Fresh Wind, Fresh Desire

By Heidi Bylsma

With Christina Motley

Fresh Wind, Fresh Desire

ISBN 9781791946319

© 2019 Heidi Bylsma
www.renewedlifementoring.com

All rights reserved. Printed in the United States of America.
No part of this book may be used or reproduced in any matter whatsoever without written permission.

Scripture quotations marked (NLT) are taken from the Holy Bible, New Living Translation, copyright © 1996, 2004, 2007 by Tyndale House Foundation. Used by permission of Tyndale House Publishers, Inc., Carol Stream, Illinois 60188. All rights reserved.

Scripture quotations marked (NIV) are taken from the Holy Bible, New International Version®, NIV®. Copyright © 1973, 1978, 1984, 2011 by Biblica, Inc.™ Used by permission of Zondervan. All rights reserved worldwide. www.zondervan.com The "NIV" and "New International Version" are trademarks registered in the United States Patent and Trademark Office by Biblica, Inc.™

Scripture quotations marked (ESV) are from the ESV® Bible (The Holy Bible, English Standard Version®), copyright © 2001 by Crossway, a publishing ministry of Good News Publishers. Used by permission. All rights reserved.

Scripture quoted by permission. Quotations designated (NET) are from the NET Bible® copyright ©1996-2016 by Biblical Studies Press, L.L.C. http://netbible.com All rights reserved.

Scripture quotations marked (HCSB) are taken from the Holman Christian Standard Bible®, Used by Permission HCSB ©1999, 2000, 2002, 2003, 2009 Holman Bible Publishers. Holman Christian Standard Bible®, Holman CSB®, and HCSB® are federally registered trademarks of Holman Bible Publishers.

Scripture quotations taken from the New American Standard Bible® (NASB),
Copyright © 1960, 1962, 1963, 1968, 1971, 1972, 1973,
1975, 1977, 1995 by The Lockman Foundation
Used by permission. www.Lockman.org

Scripture quotations taken from the Amplified® Bible (AMP),
Copyright © 2015 by The Lockman Foundation
Used by permission. www.Lockman.org

Scripture quotations taken from the New Heart English Bible (NHEB) are in the public domain. See http://studybible.info/version/NHEB for more information.

Dedications

Since 2001, I have had the blessing and privilege of enjoying the godly mentoring influence of Judy Halliday, the founder (1975) of Thin Within. Judy personifies grace itself. I dedicate this, what I consider to be my life's work, to Judy Halliday. Thank you, dear sister, for your initial invitation to join you in the writing of *Thin Within* and the *Rebuilding God's Temple Workbook Series*. Thank you for your friendship, your love, your grace, and your patience. Without you, I wouldn't have dared to dream! Your fingerprints are all over my life and the material between these covers.

For Barb Raveling. You, dear sister in the Lord, gave me a glimpse of how radically life changing and transformative "renewing the mind" can be. Thank you for your faithfulness to the work God has called you to complete. Without your influence in my life, I can't imagine where I would be today. These tools have helped me make it through marriage challenges, health crises, empty nest, moving, losing my church family (gaining a new one) and so much more!

Heidi Bylsma

To the Lord Jesus Christ, the lover of our souls, who has made a way for us to find peace and freedom in our journeys away from strongholds and toward His own heart. To Heidi, my dear friend, coach and prayer partner who Jesus has used in the most beautiful ways to lead me to the freedom Jesus offers me. To all of my dear and precious sisters in Christ who have opened their hearts and invited me to walk with them and learn from them along their journeys.

Christina Motley

"...be transformed by the renewing your mind..." Romans 12:2

INTRODUCTION

*So, whether you eat or drink, or whatever you do,
do all to the glory of God.*

1 Corinthians 10:31 (ESV)

Do you wonder if you will *ever* be at peace with food, your body, and eating? God never intended for food to *torment* His people. Rather, He desires that food and eating be a *blessing!*

Welcome to *Fresh Wind, Fresh Desire*. Here, you will discover a renewed wind blowing upon a time-tested technique—the program since 1975 that has been and continues to be called *Thin Within*. This "conscious eating" and Spirit-led approach honors the Lord with our eating, drinking and all we do.[1] More than merely one of many strategies employed to lose unwanted weight, Thin Within is a "discipleship" program, deepening our spiritual roots. In these pages, you will discover that the power of the Lord of the Universe is your primary source of strength!

As you apply Thin Within principles shared again here in *Fresh Wind, Fresh Desire*, you will release excess weight and experience a healthy, peaceful relationship with your body and with food. Your thinking, desires, *and* body will change as your mind is renewed with truth that will transform you from within![2]

Since 1975, Thin Within participants have experienced success by adopting effective tools and transforming strategies. Many of these resources are now consolidated in this study so that groups, individuals, young, old, retired, and students will experience victory with a new presentation. Years later, they continue to enjoy *staying* that size!

You *can* break free from overeating, a poor body image, habitual hopping on the bathroom scale, and beliefs that fuel unwanted feelings and behaviors. Reaching and maintaining a healthy size is an added benefit to an increased intimacy with God. We trust the Holy Spirit will breathe His fresh wind into your life and a foundation of fresh desire will arise!

You can savor the twenty-four lessons over twelve weeks, completing two lessons each week, or use eight weeks, with three assignments each week. Flexibility of this material also allows for a compact six or four-week format. An appendix is included with suggestions for leading a small group through *Fresh Wind, Fresh Desire*.

A Word about "Renewing the Mind"

In this workbook, we make reference to "mind renewal strategies." This is not a pop-psychology term but is found in the Word of God. Our theme verse is Romans 12:2 which tells us plainly that we can be transformed by God! How? Is it by keeping boundaries for my eating? By bible study and prayer? **We submit that while daily bible study and prayer are vital for the health**

---

[1] 1 Corinthians 10:31
[2] Romans 12:2

© 2019 Heidi Bylsma, www.renewedlifementoring.com. All rights reserved. Printed in the United States of America. No part of this book may be used or reproduced in any matter whatsoever without written permission.

of every Christian, these practices alone may not necessarily be the same as <u>renewing our minds in a way that God will use to transform us.</u> For instance, how many of us have filled in blanks in our bible study guide only to realize our hearts were disengaged and our "study" was little more than an intellectual exercise? How many of us take time to pray and wonder where our thoughts went for 15 minutes while we struggled to connect with God? Lists of tasks we need to do for the day or what we wish we had done during the day all clamor for attention. Have we *listened* to Him in prayer?

Therefore, we ask you to consider that *truly* renewing your mind will be the key turning the lock to your freedom. Not merely reading through the bible in a year. Not merely keeping the ACTS format for your prayers.

Prayer is speaking to God as a friend, but it is also *listening* to Him. He speaks through His Word. He also speaks directly to us by His Holy Spirit. Jesus tells us in John 16:13 that the Spirit will guide us into all truth. As we listen to the Lord, he will impress upon our hearts truth unique and specific to our lives.[3]

Because of this, our focus in *Thin Within: Fresh Wind, Fresh Desire* will be less on food or weight and more about the heart. We fix our eyes not on what is seen, but on what is unseen, for what is seen is temporary and what is unseen is eternal.[4] What is seen *will change*, but only as our hearts stop bowing to strongholds that have been erected over our years of turning to food for reasons other than physical hunger.

The tools we share in these pages will bring the Word home to your heart. You will discover what Jesus meant when he said "My sheep *listen* to my voice.[5] Those who employ the tools we teach , such as developing a God List, PraiseFest, Lessons Learned, What is True?, Big T and little t truths, Observations and Corrections, Victory List, Truth Journal, etc., have experienced breakthroughs, broken free, and are seeing the transformation that God has promised in His Word! **YOU can be among them!**

Who Are We?

Judy Halliday – Founding Thin Within in 1975, Judy, with her business partner, Joy Imboden Overstreet, pioneered the "intuitive eating" movement. Between 1975 and 1985, Thin Within workshops met in basements and libraries throughout the United States and Canada. In 1985, Thin Within workshops began to convene in churches. Judy's wisdom is found in these books: *Hunger Within, Thin Within, Raising Fit Kids in a Fat World, HEAL—Healthy Eating Abundant Living*, and our *Thin Within Rebuilding God's Temple Workbook Series*, which have transformed lives worldwide.

Heidi Bylsma – In 2001 Judy invited Heidi to collaborate on the writing of the *Thin Within* book and early versions of Thin Within's "Rebuilding God's Temple" workbook series. In 2006 and 2007, Heidi released 100 pounds using the Thin Within principles. Heidi has written at the Thin Within blog (thinwithin.org), shared in webinars, retreats and conferences, in Sound Cloud digital files, YouTube Channel videos, coaching, and Facebook study groups.

---

[3] John 16:13
[4] 2 Corinthians 4:18
[5] John 10:27

© 2019 Heidi Bylsma, www.renewedlifementoring.com. All rights reserved. Printed in the United States of America. No part of this book may be used or reproduced in any matter whatsoever without written permission.

Christina Motley, a victorious Thin Within participant, has provided extensive creative, editing, and prayer support. Together, Christina and Heidi have had the privilege and pleasure of walking with dozens of small coaching group participants through 10-week studies of *Thin Within: Fresh Wind, Fresh Desire*. For more information about our coaching group option and videos to correspond with this curriculum, please visit **https://www.thinwithin.org/fwfd/** (see appendix for more details).

Our Other Team Members are an integral part of our ministry. Leading the way behind the scenes, Joe Donaldson, the Director of Thin Within, is our shepherd, pastor, and voice of reason. Pam Donaldson, a seasoned Thin Within group leader at Southeast Christian Church in Louisville, Kentucky, supports group members and leaders around the world.

To all of these wonderful folks and to those who partnered with us in prayer through this project, we extend a most heart-felt praise to our God. We thank Him so much for you.

We hope you will visit us at our website: **http://www.thinwithin.org**. Subscribe to our newsletter to keep apprised of new online classes and other exciting announcements.

Heidi Bylsma and the Thin Within Team

© 2019 Heidi Bylsma, www.renewedlifementoring.com All rights reserved. Printed in the United States of America. No part of this book may be used or reproduced in any matter whatsoever without written permission.

LESSON 1

Scripture

Blessed are those whose strength is in you, whose hearts are set on pilgrimage.

Psalm 84:5 (NIV)

Let's Go!

What are your thoughts as you begin this adventure? What are your hopes for the time you spend in these pages and beyond? Do you have ambivalence about what is ahead? Please use the space below to write your response as a prayer to God.

_____

_____

_____

_____

A Word as You Begin Your Journey...

We boldly assert that God created us with signals of hunger and satisfaction to direct when and how much we should eat. We will encourage you that, by eating this way, you will experience a new buoyancy in your faith, but also success in melting down to your natural God-given size. We are excited about this approach.

BUT...

Thin Within and *Fresh Wind, Fresh Desire* do <u>not</u> assert that a person is ungodly, sinning or even less spiritual if they choose another means for managing their relationship with food.

God leads each of us uniquely and specifically. The last thing we want to do s provide yet another topic to divide the Church of God! So, before we get started, we want to ask you to dive into a very interesting chapter of Scripture.

Romans 14 was written by the Apostle Paul to the Roman Christians and teaches that the level of their spirituality is not demonstrated by their eating (or not) or what day they celebrate religious holidays or gather with other believers.

Please summarize or paraphrase the verses from the New Living Translation of the Bible below each quoted passage:

...One person believes it's all right to eat anything. But another believer with a sensitive conscience will eat only vegetables. **Those who feel free to eat anything must not look down on those who**

don't. *And those who don't eat certain foods must not condemn those who do, for God has accepted them. Who are you to condemn someone else's servants? Their own master will judge whether they stand or fall. And with the Lord's help, they will stand and receive his approval. ~ Romans 14:2-4 (NLT)*

_____

_____

_____

_____

So why do you condemn another believer? Why do you look down on another believer? Remember, we will all stand before the judgment seat of God. ~ Romans 14:10 (NLT)

_____

_____

_____

_____

Yes, each of us will give a personal account to God. So let's stop condemning each other. Decide instead to live in such a way that you will not cause another believer to stumble and fall. ~ Romans 14:12, 13 (NLT)

_____

_____

_____

_____

I know and am convinced on the authority of the Lord Jesus that no food, in and of itself, is wrong to eat. But if someone believes it is wrong, then for that person it is wrong. ~ Romans 14: 14 (NLT)

_____

_____

_____

_____

For the Kingdom of God is not a matter of what we eat or drink, but of living a life of goodness and peace and joy in the Holy Spirit. ~ Romans 14:17 (NLT)

_____

_____

_____

_____

We hope that you join us in concluding that no matter what we think about other eating plans, diets, and exercise programs, it is not something to criticize or judge others about.

Without further ado, then, let's get rolling!

To Release Weight...

During our time together, we will connect with marvelous truth about our God, ourselves and how well our bodies function. Our God created us fearfully and wonderfully with signals that help us to know when to eat and when to stop.[6] He makes no mistakes. When we listen, respond appropriately and go to God to have all our other needs met, we "release" any extra weight we may carry and experience peace with food, eating, and our bodies. In fact, often this change in our physical bodies comes about only as we relinquish our thoughts, minds, emotions, circumstances and situations to Him. Surrendering our unmet needs to our Mighty God enables us to be free from using overeating (or other coping mechanisms) to numb the pain we may feel. We experience a lightening of our emotional *and* physical loads. We begin to experience "weight free living!"

> ...no matter what we think about other eating plans, diets, and exercise programs, it is not something to criticize or judge others about.

Here is our first challenge for you as you start this journey: Beginning now, allow yourself to be physically hungry before any morsel crosses your lips. Sound impossible? With the strength our God provides, you can do it! You will discover food tastes more wonderful than it ever has before! Many of us can't recall when we last experienced honest-to-goodness hunger. As we prayerfully invite God to show us what true physical hunger feels like, He *will* answer.

Are you resolved to wait for true physical hunger before eating the next time? _____

The stomach is located just below our sternum (the chest bone, where the ribs come together above the midsection) and a bit to the left of center. As we hone in on what we sense in that location, we will master physical hunger.

Some signals for physical hunger are the following:

- An emptiness that isn't entirely unpleasant.

- An aching or gnawing sensation in your stomach.

- A stabbing sensation in your stomach.

_____

[6] Psalm 139:13,14

© 2019 Heidi Bylsma, www.renewedlifementoring.com. All rights reserved. Printed in the United States of America. No part of this book may be used or reproduced in any matter whatsoever without written permission.

Those who have a lot of weight to release may find it takes many hours to experience true physical hunger. Also, the larger our last meal, the longer it may take to arrive at physical hunger or, what we in call, "0" (zero). (We will talk more about the Thin Within hunger scale in Lesson 5.)

A good strategy is to busy yourself with other tasks until true physical hunger insists on having your attention. Once you arrive at a "0," enjoy a modest portion of whatever food you prefer. We will address the benefits of using discernment later. At first, we suggest you serve yourself about half the portion size you usually do. When eaten slowly enough, it might be surprising how little food it takes to satisfy! For now, just

> Many people are surprised to hear that a growl or gurgle is *not* a definitive hunger signal and may not accompany legitimate hunger. In fact, a growl or gurgle often indicates our bodies are digesting a *previous* meal!

know that your stomach is about the size of a fist and that is about the amount of food it will take to satisfy physical hunger. Never fear! You can eat again the next time you reach a "0." Jot down your thoughts and any observations about physical hunger you experience today.

___

___

___

To Do Before You Get Started

As you begin this journey into "conscious eating," ask the Lord to grant you a deep conviction that this approach is His will for you right now. While you are going through this workbook, you will want to be committed not to play with a diet simultaneously. Participants who don't make a clean break from diets end up struggling a lot during the time they are involved in *Fresh Wind, Fresh Desire*. Pray and ask Him to show you the blessings found by following these principles with your whole heart,

Respond

What questions might you ask God as you begin this journey? What do you hope to learn or know as we walk this path?

___

___

___

LESSON 2

Scripture

Glorify the Lord with me;
let us exalt his name together.

Psalm 34:3 (NIV)

Feast on the Word

Look up these passages in your Bible. Summarize the common principle or, if you want to be creative, use the first-person voice to restate each verse. (For instance, if the verse says "For God so loved the world that He gave His only Son…" you might want to write "I have loved you and this entire world so much that I have given My One and Only Son…") What does God say to you through these passages?

Romans 8:5-6   2 Corinthians 4:18   Colossians 3:1-2   Hebrews 12:2   Hebrews 3:1

_____

_____

_____

_____

Which of the following "concepts" are eternal—of the Spirit? Which are temporary or of the flesh? **Circle** the things in the list below that are eternal in nature. **Underline** the things that are temporal. Leave blank the ones you aren't sure about.

Honesty	Love for God	My weight	Humility
What I eat	My pants size	My physical fitness	Character
Worship	House	Praise	Forgiveness
Marriage	Being "Buff"	Stretch marks	God's Sovereignty

Expanding Our View of God

Let's deepen our understanding of God by exploring His character more fully—His provision, His grace, His power, His wisdom, His goodness…all of the attributes that make our God who He is.

Read Psalm 36:5-10 (we use the English Standard Version for designing this exercise). Use the chart provided below. Based on this passage, what is God like and what does he do for His people? List your observations in the chart provided. Some of your answers will be placed in the "What God is Like" column. Other answers will be placed in the "What He Does for People" column. You may have some answers that are in both columns. There are also some rectangles that will be left blank, too. The fourth column is for you to record what the Lord wants you to believe based on what you see. Some are partly done for you to help you get the hang of it. Complete those with the word(s) that comes from the verse referenced:

Verse From Psalm 36:5-10	What God is Like	What He Does for People	What He Wants me to Believe
Vs. 5	His _____ is steadfast.		
Vs. 5	He is F_____.		
Vs. 6			
Vs. 6			
Vs. 7		He gives refuge in the _____ _____ _____.	

To Release Weight...

Our wise and wonderful Lord and King has created a marvelous system for achieving and maintaining a healthy, God-given size. He has designed our bodies with distinct signals for thirst, tiredness, sickness, and to signal that we have our hands on a hot surface. We respond to all of these signals intuitively. When we have dieted or overeaten in the past, we may have ignored our body's God-given hunger/satisfied signals. That is why these signals may not be crystal clear right now. Given enough time, however, eating can become intuitive once again as we get to know and respond to our hunger and satisfied signals. As we remain prayerful and patient, our hunger/satisfied signals will become clearer. Hopefully, you are already getting acquainted with "0"—physical hunger.

Today, continue welcoming physical hunger before eating. Additionally, begin to explore and respect your body's "enough" signal. "Enough" is not "full." It is *physical* satisfaction. When you

> **Our wise and wonderful Lord and King has created a marvelous system for achieving and maintaining a healthy, God-given size.**

have had "just enough," the discomfort from hunger is gone, but you won't be uncomfortable from *overeating* either, with food pressing against the walls of your stomach. In Thin Within, we call that place of "just enough" a "5." In fact, if you were to pop up from the table and do jumping jacks after eating to a place of "just enough," a "5," or "satisfied," you could do so without any ill effects of heartburn or discomfort. (We will talk more about the hunger scale in Lesson 5.)[7]

What does physical satisfaction feel like? One participant described it as feeling like "nothing." When asked to elaborate, he said the sensation of hunger was gone—there was no longer the discomfort of an empty stomach—but there also was no sensation of having eaten too much. It is a "just enough" sensation.

As you experiment with "No longer hungry," "Just Enough," or "5," as your stopping place today, jot down your thoughts, discoveries and questions. Again, enjoy whatever food you choose, tossing aside dieting rules and legalism of the past!

_____

_____

_____

_____

Spend some time adding to your observations from Lesson 1 about eating only when you are at "0."

Respond

Consider the passages we studied today about what God is like and what He does for people… and the subsequent truths that He wants you to believe. What new thinking can you incorporate into your life? What else is on your heart today? If you like, you can answer this question as a prayer to God, using the space provided.

_____

_____

_____

_____

---

[7] Some people find greater clarity when, instead of the hunger scale of 0 to 5, they ask themselves these questions: Am I hungry? Am I no longer hungry? Am I not yet hungry?

© 2019 Heidi Bylsma, www.renewedlifementoring.com. All rights reserved. Printed in the United States of America. No part of this book may be used or reproduced in any matter whatsoever without written permission.

LESSON 3

Scripture

Jesus looked at them and said, "With man this is impossible, but with God all things are possible."

Matthew 19:26 (NIV)

Give it Some Thought

Our God is intimately acquainted with each one of us, inviting us to step into a greater story than just changing our size by dieting. Instead of fixating on **my** food, **my** will, **my** way, **my** size, **my** weight—my, my, my, my, my—let's take our eyes off of "me, myself, and I" and fix them steadfastly on our great God. As we do this, we find the impossible really *is* possible. The fear that we experienced in our dieting and compulsive exercising days dissolves. The obsession with points, calories, and pounds gained or lost may have *seemed* to strengthen our resolve when we dieted (*did* it, though?), but now we are *free*!

> **Our God is intimately acquainted with each one of us, inviting us to step into a greater story than just changing our size by dieting.**

With *FWFD*, I change my focus from how miserable *I* am, how overweight *I* am, how deprived *I* am, to how wonderful, kind, powerful, and loving my Lord and Savior, King and God is! I humble myself and exalt Him. Instead of a pity party when I am down, I have a praise party! It's hard to grab for food outside the boundaries that He has given me when I celebrate that God is King and I am His humble servant. This mindset will transform our journeys, thinking this way is not natural for us. We *can* train ourselves to think this way.

But, you say:

"I have been here before."

"I lost some weight, but I couldn't keep it off."

"How could I lose weight without dieting?"

"I did Thin Within (or other conscious eating program) before and it didn't work for me then, so why should it now?"

> **It's hard to grab for food outside of the boundaries that He has given me when I celebrate that God is King and I am His humble servant.**

Do these (or similar) thoughts bombard your mind? If so, you aren't alone. This time, however, we are going to take these thoughts captive with divine weapons capable of bringing down strongholds![8] We will live like "more-than-conquerors" in Christ.[9] Let's put on the full armor of God and take our stand against our flesh and the Enemy of our souls.[10]

In fact, all of these statements, may reflect what we call "**little t truths**."

"little t truths" and "Big T Truths"

A "**little t truth**" is something true in our *experience* as we look *back* over the *past*. (Sometimes little t truths can be in our present circumstances, but typically they refer to a *past* event.)

> **What *was* true in the past doesn't predict or define what is true *now*.**

Because little t truths actually happened to us in the **past**, we know *they are* true. This is the tricky part, though. What *was* true in the past doesn't predict or define what is true *now*. But if we give what happened in the past the power to define us going forward or to determine what will happen now and in the future, it has become a lie wrapped up inside a fact *from the past*. **Nothing from our past has the right to define us.** God reserves that right for only Him!

Instead of putting stock in what may have happened before as a good predictor of what will happen, now, let's be intentional to put "little t truths" in perspective and look at each in light of God's "Big T Truths." **"Big T Truth" is truth according to our God.** *It answers the question:*

"What would God say about that?"

Whatever the answer is to that question, *that* is the "Big T Truth" and what we want to believe! Let's look at an example:

> "Every time I have lost weight in the past I have gained it back."
> (This implies that this time won't be any different.)

Many begin FWFD spouting this "little t truth." These folks feel stuck before they start because they think that this "little t truth"—that they have gained the weight back in the past—defines what will happen now. **But this "little t truth" doesn't have the right to define what will happen going forward! We don't have to give it that kind of power!** To think it will be a reliable predictor of what will happen in the future because it is something that happened previously, is to base my life, my thinking, my actions on an assumption that this time will be like all the rest in the past.

---

[8] 2 Corinthians 10:3-5
[9] Romans 8:37
[10] Ephesians 6:10-18

© 2019 Heidi Bylsma, www.renewedlifementoring.com. All rights reserved. Printed in the United States of America. No part of this book may be used or reproduced in any matter whatsoever without written permission.

But it is believing a lie!

The more I tell myself something, the more I am likely to believe it and think it is true…even though it isn't. The past has no power over me now, unless I give it that power! Lies are often wrapped in little t truths from my past experience. Because they are "true"—they really happened to me before—I tend to think that the lie wrapped up inside of them is true, too. But I am not bound by the "truth" from my past! In fact, we don't *want* to give our past experiences (little t truths) that kind of power!

> **The past has no power over me now, unless I give it that power!**

What does God say about this little t truth—that I have always gained the weight back before (truth), so now I will as well?

The Lord God Almighty applies His strength, His wisdom, and His resurrection power into our lives **right** *now*.

The Holy Spirit, resident inside all believers in the Lord Jesus Christ, will guide us into all truth.[11] So, I want to prayerfully sit with the Lord and ask Him to show me what He says about my belief that I will gain the weight back once I lose it because I have in the past. He tells me that, as I surrender to him, hour by hour, as I keep my eyes riveted on Him instead of on the scale or on what I hope to get from food, I will experience victory not just in letting go of unhealthy extra weight, but in sustaining and maintaining my new healthy size.

We call this the "**Big T Truth**" and it is bigger and more powerful than the "little t truths." **None of our "little t truths" get to dictate what happens next.** Only God's "Big T Truths" have that power unless we *give* that power to our "little t truths." But, if we choose to keep our eyes on the Lord and welcome and believe Him for His leading, His influence, and His power in our lives, we will discover His "Big T Truth" will trump any "little t truths" that we may have allowed to defeat us —previously!

We want to tell ourselves the Big T Truth—Truth from God's perspective—over and over again so that we will believe it. We believe what we tell ourselves. We act on what we believe. So, telling myself God's view of things will help me to believe godly truth and to make godly choices!

Feast on the Word

> *Since you died with Christ to the elemental spiritual forces of this world,*
> *why, as though you still belonged to the world,*
> *do you submit to its rules:*
> *"Do not handle! Do not taste! Do not touch!"?*
> *These rules, which have to do with things*
> *that are all destined to perish with use,*
> *are based on merely human commands and teachings.*
> *Such regulations indeed have an appearance of wisdom,*
> *with their self-imposed worship, their false humility*

---

[11] John 16:13

and their harsh treatment of the body,
but they lack any value in restraining sensual indulgence.

Colossians 2:20-23 (NIV)

What is true about the "rules" referenced in this passage? Read this passage again, thinking about dieting rules you are familiar with.[12] Write your observations here:

_____

_____

_____

_____

Based on Colossians 2:20-23 we want to urge you to cast off the rules of this world!

To Release Weight....

Many people think certain *foods* make them gain weight. What if it isn't the food that is fattening, so much as the rather large portions of the foods that we eat? The belief that some foods are "virtuous" and others are not is perpetuated by diets that tell us what we can and cannot eat. Can you think of foods that you were "forbidden" from eating when you were dieting because it was thought that the **food** "was fattening?" We want to let go of dieting rules *forever* and experience the freedom that God has in mind for us."

> ...in Mark 7:19, Jesus declared all foods "clean." No food is inherently evil!

Eating *any* food in excess of our body's requirements for fuel is what causes us to gain weight. Even if it is salad! There is absolutely nothing wrong with *any* food in moderation (unless you have an allergy or a health condition that indicates otherwise). Do you find this hard to believe? Is there a "little t truth" operating in your life that says "Eating sweets (fried foods, etc.) makes me fat"? If that is a little t truth operating in your life, then you may have gained weight in the past when you have eaten that particular food and so you reason you must refrain from eating it now. Some foods *do* pack a bigger energy wallop than other foods. If we don't slow down while we eat, we won't sense that it may take fewer bites of an "energy-dense" food to satisfy us and find that we have over-eaten. And have you ever noticed that what is often referred to as "junk food," in our dieting jargon, includes the very foods that we *crave* the most? And similarly, have you noticed that what diets call "healthy food" are typically the foods we avoid (unless someone twists our arms)?

Today, continue to enjoy eating when you are physically hungry and stopping when you reach that point of "just enough." Today, however, dare to enjoy *any* food you desire (truly!) in modest

---

[12] We recognize that the context of this passage was not modern-day dieting. However, principles can be gleaned that *do* apply and that is what we hope you will consider.

© 2019 Heidi Bylsma, www.renewedlifementoring.com. All rights reserved. Printed in the United States of America. No part of this book may be used or reproduced in any matter whatsoever without written permission.

portions, but do so only when you are hungry. No food is off limits[13]. We will discuss discernment in future lessons, but today, dare to enjoy any food you desire within the parameters of God-given physical hunger and satisfaction. Consider that in Mark 7:19, Jesus declared all foods "clean." **No food is inherently evil!**

How do you feel about the thought of enjoying a food you have previously avoided due to a diet you have been on? We do encourage you to be especially prayerful, eat slowly and be sensitive to the sensations that indicate your stomach has received enough food. Evaluate if you need to tell yourself the truth about any food before you reintroduce it back into your life. If you prepare your mind by exposing lies you believe about specific foods, you won't fall into the trap many tend to fall into. Often, the first time we eat foods that we avoided previously, we get so excited that we overdo it. Tell yourself as you begin eating that you can enjoy this food in moderation and that you can have more when you get a hunger signal again. In this way, even in the presence of the most tempting "treat" (another diet word we prefer to leave behind) you will stop eating when you have had "just enough."

Write your thoughts here:

_____

_____

_____

_____

Continue to add to your thoughts about physical hunger and physical satisfaction from Lessons 1 and 2.

Respond

How do you feel about what you have studied today? Consider writing your thoughts as a prayer to the Lord.

_____

_____

_____

_____

_____

_____

---

[13] Please follow the recommendations of your medical team.

© 2019 Heidi Bylsma, www.renewedlifementoring.com All rights reserved. Printed in the United States of America. No part of this book may be used or reproduced in any matter whatsoever without written permission.

LESSON 4

Scripture

*And I am sure of this,
that he who began a good work in you
will bring it to completion at the day of Jesus Christ.*

Philippians 1:6 (ESV)

Recognizing "little t truth" and "Big T Truth"

Let's distinguish "little t truths," from "Big T Truths" and, make a point of identifying any blatant lies, too. Recall from Lesson 3 that **"little t truths" have happened in our past** (the "t" part of the label), **but they won't** *necessarily* **be true going forward** (the "little" part of the label). **"Big T Truths" are** *always* **true and** *always* **trump "little t truths." This is truth according to our sovereign God.**

> **"Big T Truths" are *always* true and *always* trump "little t truths."**

> **But God is still God and He is the only reliable source of Truth. He offers us power to defeat sin in our lives.**

Circle whether each of the following is a "little t truth," God's "Big T Truth," or LIE if it applies. Remember "little t truths" may have been true in our experience, but when taken in context with the power God has to change our lives (His "Big T Truth"), they don't carry much clout. Let's do the first three together.

1) I like food too much to be able to really eat less.

little t   BIG T   Lie

To analyze this statement, let's dissect it a bit. Notice that it has two parts: a.) I like food too much and b.) I won't be able to eat less. Part a.) *may* actually be true, but part b.) is *an assumption about now and the future based on the **past**.* It is ***predictive***. It is based on the truth that I like food, which I *do* know is true. "I ***can't*** eat less because I like food too much" is a lie, however. I **_am_** able to eat less. I *may* need to renew my mind about eating less before I actually experience it, it may be **hard,** but I **can** eat less. No one is forcing me to eat!

God's "Big T Truth" is exceedingly more powerful than your history! The chains have fallen off of countless Thin Within and FWFD participants even after loads of false starts and stops, believing lies and letting "little t truths" carry too much sway. #1 is, at its heart, a LIE. The **Big T Truth** revealed in Scripture is you can do all things through Christ Who strengthens you![14]

---

[14] Philippians 4:13

© 2019 Heidi Bylsma, www.renewedlifementoring.com. All rights reserved. Printed in the United States of America. No part of this book may be used or reproduced in any matter whatsoever without written permission.

Lies	little t truths	Big T Truths
Source is Satan	Source is our past or current experience	Source is God
Never true	True in the past or possibly in the present	Always true
Answers: "What does the enemy want me to believe?"	Answers: "What does my **experience** have to say about that?" (Assumes what has **been** will happen **now** or in the **future**. Experience is **never** a reliable indicator of what God says is true.)	Answers "What does God have to say about that?"
May be obvious when considered	Is rarely obvious as being anything but true	May seem impossible, but God is in the business of "impossible!"

Often the lies we believe – like thinking that we **can't** possibly eat less – seem true because of our *experience*, in this case knowing that I have liked and do like food a lot. If I didn't, I wouldn't eat so much. But God is still God and He is the only reliable source of Truth. He offers us power to defeat sin in our lives because Jesus conquered sin at the cross. He has given us a Spirit of love, power, and self-discipline.[15] If we have never seen the Spirit active in our lives, it doesn't mean He doesn't exist or isn't living in you. Let's be sure to scrutinize the thoughts that have held us captive in light of the truth of God's Word and His Holy Spirit!

Here's another one:

2) No matter what has come before, I know God can transform me from the inside out.

    little t   BIG T   Lie

In light of God's power provided to you, it doesn't matter how long you have struggled with food and eating. **He is at work in you right now** and He promises to complete the work He has begun.[16] This is a "Big T Truth" reflective of what God wants you to believe about food,

> …we will experience transformation that starts deep inside and penetrates outward, changing our bodies as well…

---

[15] 2 Timothy 1:7
[16] Philippians 1:6

your body, and eating. "And when we fail, God is always there to pick us up. He will continue walking with us until we have our ultimate freedom."[17]

3) I have never experienced freedom in my eating before.   little t   BIG T   Lie

This is a classic little t truth because perhaps it *is* true...maybe I have never **yet** experienced freedom in my eating...but by saying this as I continue to press on in my journey is to imply:

"...therefore, I will *never* experience freedom."

Do you see how what is really true in my *past* is being given the right to define me going forward? It may be only implied, but we urge you to notice these kinds of thoughts, too. Kick them out! They don't belong! Lies about what WILL happen in the future because of what has happened in my PAST are still LIES. If we recognize the power of God's "Big T Truth," we know it TRUMPS the "little t truth" and with God anything is possible![18]

Got the hang of it? Now it's your turn. Circle the correct label for each statement and write beneath the statement why you answered the way you did. For an additional challenge, locate a scripture reference to support your answer.

4) This is too hard for me. (Hint: This one follows the pattern of #3.)

    little t   BIG T   Lie

5) I can do all things through Christ (including learn how to eat less and enjoy it!).

    little t   BIG T   Lie

6) Even if I am successful for a while, I might fail in the end and gain all the weight back. Why should I try?

    little t   BIG T   Lie

7) Even if I mess up, I know if I am patient and hang in there, God will show me victory!

    little t   BIG T   Lie

8) In order to lose the weight, I will have to exercise a ton and eliminate certain foods.

    little t   BIG T   Lie

9) I struggle to see things through.   little t   BIG T   Lie

10) I sabotage myself often.   little t   BIG T   Lie

11) I have no self-control when it comes to eating.   little t   BIG T   Lie

---

[17] Hunger Within, page 47
[18] Matthew 19:26

12) God loves me less when I don't stay faithful.[19]   little t   BIG T   Lie

In the days ahead, we will become experts at recognizing lies and "little t truths" when we speak them to ourselves. We will begin to replace these thoughts with God's glorious "BIG T truths." We will use several tools to change our thinking and, as we do, we will experience transformation that starts deep inside and penetrates outward, changing our bodies as well!

To get a jumpstart on this process, invite God now to show you if you believe any lies that are standing in the way of experiencing the hope HE intends for you to experience. Jot them in the space provided below:

_____

_____

_____

_____

Now, ask the Lord Jesus through His Spirit to impress upon your heart what HE has to say about each of the lies or little t truths that you wrote above. What HE says is the "Big T Truth." Jot down a Big T Truth to refute each of the lies and little t truths. Put a line through each of the lies and little t truths as you write the corresponding Big T Truth on the lines below:

_____

_____

_____

_____

If you feel like it is difficult to identify the lies, don't be discouraged. This is a process—really, a way of life—for all of us. Let's invite Him to show us where we need to believe Him more completely, more accurately, more truthfully, and let's ask Him to open our eyes to what is ahead for us in this amazing journey. It is about so much more than your body or a change in your pants size! These blessings are minuscule compared to what God intends for you on this journey.

---

[19] Answers: 4) LIE, 5) T, 6) t, 7) T, 8) LIE, 9) t, 10) t, 11) LIE – see Galatians 5:22-23, 12) LIE

© 2019 Heidi Bylsma, www.renewedlifementoring.com All rights reserved. Printed in the United States of America. No part of this book may be used or reproduced in any matter whatsoever without written permission.

What do you think?

What do you think about the "Big T" and "little t" truths in your life? Take a moment to ask God to give you wisdom to recognize lies and "little t truths" in your life so you can counter anything you need to with God's "Big T Truth."

_____

_____

_____

_____

To Release Weight

Continue to select any food you enjoy between the parameters of your physical hunger, "0," and physical satisfaction, "5." In the space below, write any additional observations, feelings, questions, and prayers you may have about this.

_____

_____

Respond

What is on your heart today?

_____

_____

_____

_____

_____

_____

_____

© 2019 Heidi Bylsma, www.renewedlifementoring.com. All rights reserved. Printed in the United States of America. No part of this book may be used or reproduced in any matter whatsoever without written permission.

LESSON 5

Scripture

Do not conform to the pattern of this world,
but be transformed by the renewing of your mind.
Then you will be able to test and approve
what God's will is—his good, pleasing and perfect will.

Romans 12:2 (NIV)

Moving Forward!

Let's think back to our dieting days. Life was black or white, pass or fail, good or bad. Each day was a success or failure depending on our weight on the scale or how much we had eaten of our allotted points, fat grams, calories, fiber, or whatever else. More often than not, the math did not work out in our favor and we were quick to condemn ourselves. We subsequently recommitted to "being good," or "threw in the towel," convinced we had failed yet another diet.

Not only this, but during our dieting days, we categorized foods into categories of "good foods" and "bad foods." When we ate the "good foods," we felt virtuous. When we ate from the "bad foods" list, *we* were bad!

And when we *did* lose weight, we proudly collected the praises of friends and family while secretly being afraid of gaining it all back. And if we gained weight again, people observed in silence and we adopted the painful label "FAILURE."

> **Changing our thinking changes our beliefs. Changing our beliefs changes our actions. Changing our actions changes our results.**

Many of us have been stuck in this cycle again and again. What is the key to breaking free? How do we find true, lasting transformation? Romans 12:2 sheds light—*the renewing of our minds* is the answer. What does "renew our minds" mean? Reading our Bibles more? Praying more? Memorizing more Scripture? No. Are you surprised to hear us say, "No"?

Of course, we recommend every participant read the Word of God and pray as well as practice the many other Christian disciplines (fasting, giving, serving, solitude, etc.). But when it comes to renewing your mind, we ask you to prayerfully consider what **God might be speaking to your heart personally if He were to sit down with you** right now, today. Does that sound too vague? If you are a believer, you have the Presence of the Spirit of God within you, to instruct you, convict you, remind you of things you have learned. While the impressions you get by asking the Lord "What are *your* thoughts about this, Lord?" aren't on par with scripture, God is remarkably practical, and you may be surprised at the kinds of "Big T Truths" he impresses on your heart.

Here are some of mine:

- When _____ (a difficult person in my life) is rude or downright mean, I don't need to let it affect my thinking *or* my eating.

- God is always at work doing a new thing in my life, including in my eating.

- The most important meal of the day for me is the one that I am hungry for.

- When I feel the need to comfort myself, the Lord, who calls Himself my Comforter, is standing by to supply the comfort I need. I can turn to Him and let HIM calm me.

In the lessons ahead, we will introduce tools that you can use to renew your mind, so your thinking will change. Changing our thinking changes our beliefs. Changing our beliefs changes our actions. Changing our actions changes our results.

What comes to mind when you think of "FAILURE?"

FAILURE

_____

_____

_____

_____

Have you ever wondered about how God views failure?

Think About It

"It is finished," Jesus said, and then breathed His last on the cross. In that moment, Satan, the enemy of all mankind thought he had won. Jesus' dejected disciples gave up everything to follow Him. All now seemed lost. Those who plotted the death of Jesus celebrated their victory. What had happened on the cross, *appeared* to be the most colossal "failure" of all time as, they reasoned, if Jesus had been the Messiah, he would have been a conquering warrior and militarily defeat Rome.

What the world saw as failure, however, was really an inconceivable, divine victory in disguise! Christ's death on the cross was the single act, which, for *all* time, ensured *all* men and women *everywhere* would have the opportunity for an eternal relationship with the God of the universe. Jesus Christ took all of our sin upon Him, so we might be credited with His righteousness.[20] Redemption! Our God IS our *great* Redeemer. This is true now and always. If He can redeem the worst, most torturous death the Roman Empire could carry out, He can certainly redeem our missteps and mistakes with eating and food. In anything and everything we might perceive as a failure, our God rises to show us His compassion[21] and His redemption.

---

[20] 2 Corinthians 5:21
[21] Isaiah 30:18

© 2019 Heidi Bylsma, www.renewedlifementoring.com. All rights reserved. Printed in the United States of America. No part of this book may be used or reproduced in any matter whatsoever without written permission.

No matter what has come before this day in your life, wait on Him. He promises not to waste a single minute. Be encouraged and know **God will use everything for His glory! He will provide new strength**[22] **and grant you ability to see that He is doing a new thing**[23]**, redeeming everything in your past.** What an amazing truth this is!

Respond to this assertion in the space below:

> **God will use everything for His glory! He will provide new strength and grant you ability to see that He is doing a new thing, redeeming *everything* in your past.**

_____

_____

_____

_____

Because our God is Redeemer, He has the ability to take every failure and transform it! Each failure becomes an opportunity for victory, equipping us with weapons of warfare to demolish strongholds[24], to experience victory, living our birthright to be more than conquerors in Christ[25]. From this vantage point, we can enjoy the freeing truth that failure is a powerful tool to teach us—all in the hands of our great, creative, redeeming God!

Think of a challenging situation you have recently faced. While difficult at the time, how did this experience deepen your faith or teach you a valuable lesson? Describe it here:

_____

_____

_____

_____

Let's renew our minds about failure!

Dieting may not have worked for us, but God is doing a new thing[26], leading us to trust Him and His design of our bodies. Let's take a look at a tool Thin Within calls the Hunger Scale.

---

[22] Isaiah 40:31
[23] Isaiah 43:19
[24] 2 Corinthians 10:4
[25] Romans 8:37
[26] Isaiah 43:19

© 2019 Heidi Bylsma, www.renewedlifementoring.com All rights reserved. Printed in the United States of America. No part of this book may be used or reproduced in any matter whatsoever without written permission.

To Release Weight – The Hunger Scale

Thin Within teaches us that our goal is to eat between a 0 (an empty stomach, physical hunger) and a 5 (a comfortably filled stomach pouch, satisfied, or "just enough"). If we eat within these parameters -- between 0 and 5 -- we will shrink down to our natural, God-given size and maintain it (see Figure 1).

If we eat between a 3 and a 7 on the hunger scale, we will maintain a larger than ideal size.

If we eat between a 5 and a 10 on the hunger scale, we will continue to get larger. A 10 is that "over the top, I must get horizontal and unbutton my pants" feeling you have when you have stuffed yourself. It is extremely uncomfortable.

Today, continue to eat between physical hunger and satisfaction (0 and 5), selecting a modest portion of foods you truly enjoy.[27] Eating slowly will help you to eat less as you will be able to notice satisfaction more readily.

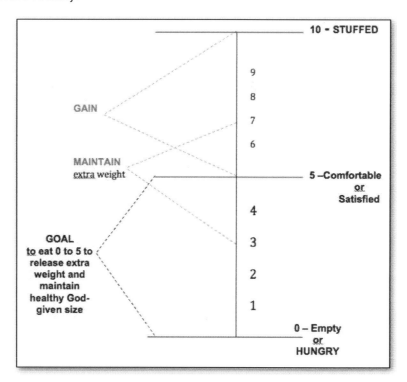

Figure 1

> **It takes about ten to twenty minutes for your stomach to signal your brain you don't need any more food.**

---

[27] For some new to conscious, intuitive eating, it can sometimes be easier to ask yourself "Am I hungry?" or "Am I not hungry?" before deciding to eat. Then, if you are hungry, as you eat, you can evaluate "Am I no longer hungry?" and "No longer hungry" can be your stopping place. Later you may be able to use the specific hunger numbers more effectively.

© 2019 Heidi Bylsma, www.renewedlifementoring.com. All rights reserved. Printed in the United States of America. No part of this book may be used or reproduced in any matter whatsoever without written permission.

When we eat too fast, we often bypass our 5 and do not realize it until our stomach finally communicates with our brain. We think, "Oops! I am at a '7'" even though we didn't intend to overeat.

Here are some strategies to slow down our eating:

- Eat everything with utensils. We tend to eat finger foods quickly.

- Use your less dominant hand. If you are right handed, use your left. If you are left handed, use your right. This helps for a few days—until you learn how to eat with your less dominant hand!

- Put your fork (or spoon) down between bites.

- Sip your beverage between each bite.

What will you do to eat more slowly this week?

_____

_____

_____

_____

Thoughts to consider:

Have you felt emotional lately as you have begun to modify your eating, staying between the boundaries of 0 and 5? Have you been more emotional than usual? Maybe you have been surprised how easily you are frustrated, irritated or reduced to tears. Many participants are surprised to hear that this is normal for many of us who have used food to numb ourselves to our emotions previously. Since we are no longer using food that way, we are likely to *feel* our emotions more keenly as we make these changes. When this happens, be encouraged and know God intends for you to be healed and to develop *healthy* coping mechanisms for whatever you are going through. Pray and search out his Word, the Bible, to seek personal encouragement straight from His heart to yours. Jot down anything you discover or wonder about:

_____

_____

_____

_____

Without including food, prayerfully generate a plan that you can follow when you feel surprisingly emotional.

_____

Respond

What has the Lord shown you today? How will you respond?

LESSON 6

Scripture

*The boundary lines have fallen for me in pleasant places;
surely I have a delightful inheritance.*

Psalm 16:6 (NIV)

Boundaries

Driving along a scenic, two-lane country road, suddenly an oncoming car pulls around a slow RV to pass, flying into our lane and coming straight for us. First, we panic, but once the danger passes, we become indignant! Life is full of boundaries we respect without question. The double yellow line down the middle of a windy canyon road reminds drivers *not* to pass. The wooden fence protects a family dog from wandering off into a forest where predators lurk. The gate at the top of the stairs protects the baby from falling and hurting himself. Boundaries guard us, protecting what is precious.

> **Boundaries guard us, protecting what is precious.**

We are familiar with boundaries because we have used them while dieting in the past. For instance, we set limits of how much food we should eat and when we should eat it. We ate "good" foods and tried to stay away from "bad" foods. We limited and counted calories, fat grams, fiber, or something similar, establishing these as "boundaries" for our eating. These kinds of boundaries may have had an appearance of wisdom at the time, but those of us who have started *Thin Within* or *Fresh Wind, Fresh Desire* right out of the dieting world, have found we had trouble maintaining them for a reason. These human-made structures often create a tendency toward obsession and self-condemnation and do nothing at all to change our hearts (Colossians 2:20-23).

In this approach, we have freedom from "good food" or "bad food" lists. God's Word teaches us not to be gluttonous or greedy.[28] God has created us fearfully and wonderfully,[29] so 0 to 5 eating is an appropriate application of Scripture. Life with God-given boundaries is all about respecting the wonderful way God has made our bodies to signal us as we eat between physical hunger and physical satisfaction – 0 and 5. There is such relief for us in this truth! Be assured you will grow in your willingness to go to God with every reason you might turn to food other than physical need. Renewing our minds will be the only means we will use to change our thinking permanently and experience the transformation we long for—from *within*.

> **We have freedom from "good food" or "bad food" lists!**

God's boundaries for His children are pleasant (Psalm 16:6). 0 to 5 eating is a delightful boundary (honest!); it is the way our bodies work naturally.

---

[28] Proverbs 23:20-21; Colossians 3:5; Ephesians 5:3
[29] Psalm 139:14

© 2019 Heidi Bylsma, www.renewedlifementoring.com All rights reserved. Printed in the United States of America. No part of this book may be used or reproduced in any matter whatsoever without written permission.

If we stay within this boundary, we will enjoy the freedom and peace to eat any food we desire, while releasing extra weight in a natural and healthy way.

What are some eating boundaries you have used in the past?

_____

_____

_____

Restate the primary boundary for what we are doing in *Fresh Wind, Fresh Desire* (think "hunger" and "satisfaction").

_____

_____

_____

More on Boundaries

Fill in the following chart as you investigate boundaries mentioned in Scripture. What is the boundary? Who established the boundary? Who benefits from the boundary? If you don't find a detailed answer in the passage, prayerfully consider it and write down what comes to mind.

Verse	Description of Boundary	Who established the boundary?	Who benefits? How?
Job 26:10			
Psalm 74:17			
Psalm 104:5-9			
Proverbs 8:27-29			

Summarize here what you have discovered, learned, or been reminded of about boundaries through the Bible study above.

_____

© 2019 Heidi Bylsma, www.renewedlifementoring.com. All rights reserved. Printed in the United States of America. No part of this book may be used or reproduced in any matter whatsoever without written permission.

To Release Weight

> **God-given boundaries protect and venerate what is prized.**

God-given boundaries protect and esteem what is prized. If you want to honor the boundary of hunger/satisfied eating, it helps to adopt guidelines or "secondary boundaries" that support awareness of your hunger level. When we put these strategies together with eating between hunger and satisfaction, they compose what we call the "Eight Keys to Conscious Eating."

Since 1975, Thin Within has taught that we can benefit by following the habits of people who stay a healthy size without dieting or exercising obsessively. Judy Halliday observed that naturally healthy-sized people practice these keys without thinking! We suggest you bathe your mealtimes in prayer to experience each key as a wonderful opportunity to glorify God.[30]

Keys to Conscious Eating[31]

1. Eat when your body is hungry.

2. Eat in a calm environment by reducing distractions.

3. Eat when sitting.

4. Eat when your body and mind are relaxed.

5. Eat and drink only the things that your body loves.

6. Pay attention only to your food while eating.

7. Eat slowly, savoring each bite.

8. Stop before your body is full.

You may recognize Keys #1 and #8 as being our primary boundary of eating 0 to 5.

We have previously asked you to follow Key #5—to eat and drink only the things that your body loves. In Lesson 5 we also asked you to slow down as you eat—Key #7. Today, continue to follow Keys 1, 5, 7, and 8. Circle them in the list above.

---

[30] 1 Corinthians 10:31
[31] Thin Within's influence on this material can't be overstated. Much of this is Judy Halliday's material, in a new presentation.

© 2019 Heidi Bylsma, www.renewedlifementoring.com All rights reserved. Printed in the United States of America. No part of this book may be used or reproduced in any matter whatsoever without written permission.

Additionally, select one of the remaining Keys you think might be helpful to you today and tomorrow. Pick one that will help you be aware of when a 5 is approaching so you don't eat past the "just enough" point. Circle it in the list and write your strategy here:

Respond

What has the Lord shown you today? How would He like you to respond?

LESSON 7

Scripture

*Do you not know that your bodies are temples of the Holy Spirit,
who is in you, whom you have received from God?
You are not your own; you were bought at a price.
Therefore honor God with your bodies.*

1 Corinthians 6:19-20 (NIV)

Your Body is God's Temple on Earth!

Our glorious, magnificent God no longer inhabits a temple or tabernacle as He did during the time of Moses and Solomon. *YOU* are His preferred dwelling place! He purchased YOU with Christ's blood![32] Write this truth in your own words:

_____

_____

_____

_____

Deep inside the minds and hearts of some of us doing the exercise above, the thought (or similar) might emerge:

> "Nope, that's not me, not *this* body! I have let this body get too heavy, too broken down, too out of shape. There is no way God would want to live in me given how poorly I have taken care of this body."

Can you identify with this thought? How?

_____

_____

_____

_____

---

[32] 1 Peter 1:18-19

© 2019 Heidi Bylsma, www.renewedlifementoring.com. All rights reserved. Printed in the United States of America. No part of this book may be used or reproduced in any matter whatsoever without written permission.

Since Lesson 3, we have recognized lies and "little t truths" and replaced them with God's "Big T Truths." Let's apply this strategy here. Hopefully you can see the above statement is a lie. Write "LIE" in big bold capital letters across the statements in the box.

Now, prayerfully welcoming God to tell us what His thoughts are about this, we listen for the Holy Spirit. This lie can be countered with God's "Big T Truth:"

> "No matter how I have treated my body, no matter what condition it is in, as a believer in the Lord Jesus Christ, God delights to have purchased and claimed my body for His use."

Circle the above statement, asterisk it, and write "TRUTH" in the margin next to the box.

Another lie many of us may believe:

> "It doesn't matter what I do. My body is mine to do with as I please."

Write "LIE" across this statement as you did with the previous lie. If we subscribe to this lie, we may resist God's will regarding our bodies and our eating.

The "Big T Truth" to apply here is:

> "I am fearfully and wonderfully made by God's own design.[33] God has purchased my body with the blood of Jesus. I belong to Him for His purposes."

As with the previous Truth, circle and asterisk this, then write TRUTH in big bold letters beside the box in the margin.

One final example is:

> God doesn't care about my food, eating or my weight.

This implies that I can eat what I want when I want without negative ramifications to my walk with God. Yet, is that true? No! The truth is, God wants me to respond to His leadership by being obedient. If he convicts me to stop eating and I continue to eat, if he convicts me that I should not start eating and I do anyway, I am rejecting his leadership. THIS is at the heart of our eating issues, not one bite too many of this or that! It is rebellious to reject his direction and to turn my back on it.

---

[33] Psalm 139:14

Responding to the "Big T Truth"

It is important that we recognize the lies and "little t truths" upon which many of our behaviors are built and diligently apply God's "Big T Truth" to them. This will affect our actions in a powerful way. We can do this by developing a habit of rejecting the lies (even out loud) and speaking the Big T Truths out loud. The more we do this, the more likely we are to truly renew our minds—to think differently—to see the transformation that Romans 12:2 promises.

What are some consequences we experience because of the belief that our body is ours to do with as we please? For example: "When I believed my body was mine to do with as I pleased, I ate all I wanted even when I was full. This caused me to be overweight and my joints ached every day."

Your turn—What consequences did you experience by believing your body was yours to do with as you pleased?

_____

_____

_____

_____

God declares that you are **His** and your physical body is for **His** beautiful purposes. How might believing—*really believing*—this Big T Truth affect you? What choices might that cause you to make?

_____

_____

_____

_____

If I believe "I am my own and I can do as I please!" then I eat just because I want to, because the food is delicious, because I feel entitled, because I feel justified, because it's a time of day when I "should" eat, etc.

If I tell myself the Big T Truth again and again, that my body belongs to God and that he has merely entrusted it to my care, I will begin to believe it. Whatever I tell myself is what I will believe. We want to drive this point home, so bear with us as we repeat it yet again: **What I believe is going to drive my actions. As I tell myself Big T Truth, I will believe them, my desires will change, and my actions will change.** I will have a mind and a tenderness to what the Lord would have me do and this will affect when I eat, why I eat, how much of it I eat and how frequently I eat. My actions will be driven by what I believe. My beliefs are formed and shaped by what I tell myself. Do you see how telling ourselves

> **Whatever I tell myself is what I will believe.**

the Big T Truth about our bodies belonging to God can radically transform our issues with food and our view of our bodies?

Here are some "Big T Truths" for you to ponder. Say each one **out loud,** then, beside each one, write the word TRUTH in big bold letters:

- I am precious to God, just as I am. _____
- My body is not my own. It belongs to God. _____
- Even before I release the extra weight and consistently eat within hunger/satisfied boundaries, *I* am *His* precious temple. _____
- I am His chosen dwelling place. _____
- He has given me His Holy Spirit who lives in me. _____
- My body is not my own; He has a purpose for me. _____
- The same resurrection power that blew the lid off Jesus' grave is present within me. _____
- God is at work in me every single day! _____

Creating Truth Cards[34]

Over the years, we have found the people who are most likely to experience breakthrough and experience lasting freedom and permanent release of their extra weight and peace with food are those who are diligent to apply Romans 12:2—they renew their minds with Truth. Truth straight out of the Word, Truth personalized from bible verses, and Truth impressed on their hearts by the Holy Spirit through listening prayer. This week, we want to *strongly* urge you to purchase some index cards—even better to get a spiral bound deck, available at an office supply store. (Alternatively, you can just do this assignment on your computer or hand-write a list.) As you continue studying this workbook and when you notice a lie or "little t truth" running through your mind, write the "Big T Truth" that counters it on an index card -- "Truth Card" -- or add it to your Truth List. The previous bulleted statements are a great place to start in creating your own deck of Truth Cards or a Truth List. Throughout this workbook, we will make suggestions about additions for your Truth Card deck. You can come up with your own as well, as God's Spirit leads and directs you.

Fill in the blanks in the following statement with a day of the week that will fit with your schedule. Please don't overlook the significance of this assignment. We will be referring to Truth Cards/Truth Lists again and again. Those who **follow** through will have a ***break*** through!

---

[34] Feel free to create a "Truth List" instead of a deck of Truth Cards. These lists can then travel with you in your phone, if you like.

© 2019 Heidi Bylsma, www.renewedlifementoring.com. All rights reserved. Printed in the United States of America. No part of this book may be used or reproduced in any matter whatsoever without written permission.

| This week, I will get some index cards or a spiral bound deck of index cards on _____ (what day this week will work for you?) and I will check this box once I have gotten them. ☐

On _____ (what day this week will work for you?) I will start writing Truths on my Truth Cards or in a Truth List, beginning with those listed above. |

Truth Cards in Action

While one suggested use of Truth Cards is to read (out loud) through them when you are tempted to eat outside of your hunger/satisfied (0 to 5) eating boundaries, we have found **the most effective use is to *prepare for your day*** by using them to "wall paper" your mind with the Truth. If five or ten minutes in the morning won't work for you, select another time of day to do this. Then read some of your Truth Cards out loud. In this way, you will engage a number of learning modalities, getting the TRUTH into your mind and heart more effectively! Looking at your cards/list you **see** the Truth. Reading the card/list out loud, forms the Truth on your lips. As you **say** the Truth, you also **hear** the Truth. You will be amazed at how doing this will renew your mind and then, when you are faced with a tempting situation, **your *renewed mind* will kick in with godly instruction.**

> **Those who follow through will have a break through!**

You will discover that, over time of renewing your mind, you will actually develop new *desires*.

For years we have practiced thinking and believing thoughts that have not served us— "little t truths" and downright lies. This has led us to turn to food for a variety of reasons other than physical need:

- to "decompress" after a stressful day.
- to find comfort.
- to celebrate.
- to deal with boredom.

What other reasons do you overeat?

- _____
- _____
- _____

© 2019 Heidi Bylsma, www.renewedlifementoring.com All rights reserved. Printed in the United States of America. No part of this book may be used or reproduced in any matter whatsoever without written permission.

To be transformed by the renewing of our minds, we will tear down the "wallpaper" that is currently pasted on the walls of our minds. We will be done with our old way of thinking and put up new "wallpaper"—God's "Big T Truth" wallpaper! We want to **think God's thoughts after him**.

We invite you to make this a priority for the next 17 lessons. How do you feel about doing that?

_____

_____

_____

_____

I will be intentional to carve out 5 to 10 minutes at least once daily

for reading my Truth Cards/Truth List.

(Please check the box if you are on board!) ☐

The best time of the day for me is likely to be

_____

A secondary time I could try is _____

To Release Weight – Evaluate Your Use of the Bathroom Scale

> **…your renewed mind will kick in with godly instruction.**

Many people wonder how often they should weigh. The answer to this is, truthfully, "It depends." Through your dieting experiences, has using the bathroom scale served you in a positive way? Has it ever helped you to lose weight on diets and keep it off? What feelings do you get when you step on the scale and how do you respond to those feelings? Are you able to use the scale as merely a tool or a reality test, every few weeks? Or do you find yourself obsessing about the numbers and hopping on the bathroom scale numerous times in a day? Take a moment and write your thoughts.

_____

_____

_____

_____

Prayerfully ask God what He wants you to do with the bathroom scale?

© 2019 Heidi Bylsma, www.renewedlifementoring.com. All rights reserved. Printed in the United States of America. No part of this book may be used or reproduced in any matter whatsoever without written permission.

Respond

What has the Lord shown you today? How would He like you to respond?

LESSON 8

Scripture

*You were taught, with regard to your former way of life,
to put off your old self, which is being corrupted by its deceitful desires;
to be made new in the attitude of your minds...*

Ephesians 4:22-23 (NIV)

The Power of Truth

The Truth will set us free.[35] This is the priceless value of abiding in Jesus' teaching. We have an opportunity to see this Truth fleshed out in our eating as we ask Him to show us His thoughts about our bodies, food, and the changes He is making in us.

More About Truth Cards

Since using Truth Cards or a Truth List can be a vital part of *permanent* transformation, here are some questions and thoughts to help you come up with Truths to create your Truth Card deck and renew your mind. Write out your answers and turn them into truths for your Truth Card deck or Truth List:

- What is true about 0 to 5 eating?
    - What benefits do I experience when I depend on my fearfully and wonderfully made body to signal when and how much to eat? What benefits, other than the physical benefit of releasing weight or maintaining a healthy size, are a part of this? How is God growing me?
    - Is life better with boundaries? Or is it worse?
    - Is more food better? Why or why not?
- Some ideas to consider:
    - 0 to 5 enables me to enjoy all things in an appropriate amount.
    - I need boundaries all the time. I am not someone who can eat whenever I want as much as I want, without it negatively impacting my life!

---

[35] John 8:32

- If my body is *not* my own to do with as I please, who **does** own my body? What implications does this Truth have?

  _____

  _____

- Based on the thoughts, questions and answers, what are some specific Truths you will include in your Truth Card deck or Truth List? Write them in the space below.

  _____

  _____

  _____

  _____

When will you add these to your Truth Card deck/Truth List? _____

(Check this box when you have done so.) ☐

Expanding our View of God

In Lesson 2, we looked up a passage and filled in a chart that answered the questions "What is God Like?" and "What Does He Do for People?" Let's do that again today. This time, you get to choose which passage you use; you can try a Psalm or a chapter in Isaiah and fill in the following chart:

Passage I Chose: _____	What God is Like	What He Does for People	What God Wants Me to Believe
Verse:			
Verse:			
Verse:			
Verse:			

We will use these charts or "God Lists" for a very important renewing of the mind activity in a later lesson. Referring to Lesson 2 and the chart above, what are your favorite truths about God from your God List? Why?

_____

_____

_____

_____

Review the Truth Cards/Truth List you already have and/or add some new Truths to your deck or Truth List. *(Check this box when you have done so.)* ☐

To Release Weight – Portion Sizes

The stomach is like a deflated balloon when it is empty. When enough food has been eaten to send the brain a "satisfied" signal, the stomach has expanded to about the size of a loosely clenched fist[36]. It will require merely a fist-sized portion of food to bring you from 0 to a 5 on the hunger scale. That's not as much food as most of us are accustomed to eating and not everyone can begin with a fist-sized portion. If a fist-sized helping is not workable yet, try cutting your serving sizes back to half or two-thirds of what you served yourself in the past. Over time, you can make additional changes.

> Eat half as much, twice as slowly, savoring it along the way, and you will land on the last bite at the same moment as you would by eating the old way, only this time you will enjoy it so much more AND your body will thank you!

One reason why this tactic is so effective is it is the last bite we so often feel "sad" about. If we eat half as much, half as fast, our brains think they got just as much enjoyment out of it…maybe more!

By two or three weeks, if your pants haven't gotten a bit looser, and you think you have been stopping at a 5, we urge you to consider reducing your portions a bit further. It could be that you might need to "refine" your 5. In Lesson 23, we discuss the "Margin of 5."

While many participants successfully avoid eating until they are at 0, it is more challenging to stop when your body signals it is at a 5.[37] It helps to slow down. Serving ourselves less food and eliminating seconds are also beneficial strategies.

---

[36] We urge you to use some of the mind renewal strategies to tell yourself the truth about eating less food. This will build a willingness in your heart and mind that may surprise you!

[37] One reason for this is because we are eager to "find" 0 so we get to eat! But looking diligently for a 5 means we have to stop eating. It is harder to "find" something we don't *want* to find!

© 2019 Heidi Bylsma, www.renewedlifementoring.com. All rights reserved. Printed in the United States of America. No part of this book may be used or reproduced in any matter whatsoever without written permission.

Verse:			
Verse:			
Verse:			
Verse:			
Verse:			
Verse:			

How do you feel about your portion sizes? Is there room to adjust? Remember, when you get hungry, you can always eat again!

___

Respond

What has the Lord shown you today? How would He like you to respond?

___

LESSON 9

Scripture

*But you are a chosen people, a royal priesthood, a holy nation,
God's special possession,
that you may declare the praises of him who called you out of darkness into his wonderful light.*

1 Peter 2:9 (NIV)

Who Are You?

Who do you believe you are? Do you believe you are who God says you are? What you believe has a direct impact on the choices you make each and every day, including choices about eating!

Think About It

Do you remember "dress up?" Cowboy boots, swagger in our step, we drawled, "Howdy!" We *were* cowboys. Heels and a fancy dress—we *glided* regally across the "ballroom" as princesses. What we wore made a difference in who we believed we were. We acted based on our belief. It was much more than pretend!

Similarly, someone whose identity is rooted in being a marathon runner acts according to this belief. She dresses, eats, reads, speaks, and does all things "running." A person who thinks of himself as a sports fan invests time, money and energy on games, statistics and social events celebrating his favorite sport. His actions reflect that being a sports fan is an important part of his identity.

Beliefs result in actions. Actions establish patterns in our lives and the patterns bring forth results.

Beliefs → Actions → Patterns → Results

God has attributed an identity to each of us. *He* tells us in the Bible who we are. When we believe what <u>He</u> says, we live, breathe, speak, play and work—***act***—like we are who *He* says we are.

Feast on the Word

In the following Scripture references, underline words that describe ***you*** as one of God's children:

> "Therefore, if anyone is in Christ, he is a new creation. The old has passed away; behold, the new has come." 2 Corinthians 5:17 (ESV)
>
> "[E]ven as he chose us in him before the foundation of the world, that we should be holy and blameless before him…." Ephesians 1:4 (ESV)
>
> "He has delivered us from the domain of darkness and transferred us to the kingdom of his beloved Son…." Colossians 1:13 (ESV)
>
> "You are the light of the world. A city set on a hill cannot be hidden." Matthew 5:14 (ESV)
>
> "[W]ho saved us and called us to a holy calling, not because of our works but because of his own purpose and grace, which he gave us in Christ Jesus before the ages began..." 2 Timothy 1:9 (ESV)
>
> "But now in Christ Jesus you who once were far off have been brought near by the blood of Christ." Ephesians 2:13 (ESV)
>
> "Therefore, we are ambassadors for Christ, God making his appeal through us." 2 Corinthians 5:20a (ESV)
>
> "[A]nd in Christ you have been brought to fullness. He is the head over every power and authority." Colossians 2:10 (NIV)
>
> "In him you also, when you heard the word of truth, the gospel of your salvation, and believed in him, were sealed with the promised Holy Spirit, who is the guarantee of our inheritance until we acquire possession of it, to the praise of his glory." Ephesians 1:13-14 (ESV)

Complete the following sentence with a list of the attributes you underlined in the verses above, then asterisk the descriptions or words that especially speak to you:

Because God has declared it to be true in His eternal, reliable Word, I am:

_____

_____

_____

_____

How might it affect your actions if you believed these things to be true? How might you treat your body differently?

___

___

___

___

Use what you wrote to create new truths in your Truth Cards/Truth List about who you are according to the Bible. For instance: "I am a new creature in Christ. I am not who I *was*. The old me is gone. The new me has come![38]" Or, "Overeating will never satisfy like fullness in Christ!" *(Check this box when you have done that.)* ☐

To Release Weight – Look and Learn[39]

> **We can't hate ourselves into positive change.**

One of the best tools we can use on our Thin Within journey is that of "Look and Learn[40]." Let's learn from every "mess up" and "failure"—even a binge! Our Great Redeemer will have His way with us. When we dieted and "messed up" by noon, we often finished the day with the train "off the rails." We condemned ourselves resulting in even more unrestrained behavior. We can't hate ourselves into positive change.

It's been said: "We have to do something different to get different results." Let's **LOOK** prayerfully and *dispassionately* at our behavior and dismantle a situation when we overate. Did we start the day tired? Did a friend hurt our feelings? Did someone surprise us with a gift of our favorite food when we had just eaten? Was our conviction wavering? Did we have a rebellious heart or did it happen unintentionally, perhaps by eating too quickly?

> **Beliefs result in actions. Actions establish patterns in our lives and the patterns bring forth results.**

Looking carefully, we note numerous decision points before we chose to break our 0 to 5 boundaries. For instance, I can eat Oreo milkshakes…they are lawful, but when I have vanilla ice cream in my freezer and Oreo cookies in the cupboard, I will have a milkshake for every single 0 to 5 meal!

Permissible, yes. But beneficial? Hardly! So, willingly and with joy, I haven't had Oreos and Vanilla ice cream in my house at the same time for a long while. When I am out and about, I am free to get a milkshake when I am at a 0.

---

[38] 2 Corinthians 5:17; Colossians 2:10
[39] Please see Appendix D for more information about Look and Learn
[40] Referred to as "Observation and Correction" in other Thin Within materials.

© 2019 Heidi Bylsma, www.renewedlifementoring.com. All rights reserved. Printed in the United States of America. No part of this book may be used or reproduced in any matter whatsoever without written permission.

Let's say for the purposes of illustration that the last time I blew past my 5 it was with home-made milkshakes. What decision points were there along the way for me?

Decision Point	What I *could* have done instead
I notice that I woke up tired and my energy is dragging the first hours of the day.	I consider this fact a red flare indicating I may be vulnerable. I anticipate the temptation and begin now renewing my mind and preparing for action.
I purchase vanilla ice cream and Oreo cookies at the store and brought them home, even though history told me it wasn't a good idea.	I can leave them at the store. By purchasing them, I make provision for the flesh (Romans 13:14)
I walk into the kitchen and get out a big glass and the blender.	Even now, I can stop and renew my mind for even 5 minutes. Usually, when I do that, I don't even WANT what-ever-it-is.
I scoop the ice cream (it isn't typically easy to do that) and begin to break up the cookies as I put the ingredients in the blender.	Even at this point, I can stop! I can put it all away or, even, throw it all away.
The milkshake is made and I start eating and/or go back for seconds and face decision points once again.	Get in the bathtub and relax to Christian music and candles or go for a walk, call a friend, journal what I am feeling, etc.

This is just a quick overview of some of the decision points and options I have along the way, but there are definitely more. At *any* point in time, I can choose to turn around, throw the milkshake away, stop eating, etc.

Let's proactively apply Big T Truth *before* temptation strikes. Each morning, we can prepare for the day ahead by wall-papering our minds with Truth, prayerfully reviewing our Truth Cards/Truth List. Renewing our minds minimizes the likelihood later in the day that we will be swept up in emotion and break our eating boundaries.

Looking at a stumble of ours provides an opportunity to see what happened. We can ask our Heavenly Daddy to show us His viewpoint.

Now, we can **learn** from it and develop a plan for next time—a plan to act differently.[41] We can learn to view each challenging situation, trial, holiday, vacation, or stressful dinner as a "training opportunity," teaching us how we can be victorious in the future. We apply God's grace to our everyday moments. God's grace in action.

LOOK: It is your turn! Picture the last time you broke your eating boundaries. What decision points preceded the event? Did you decide to turn away from God's leadership and choose to overeat intentionally? When? What emotions, circumstances, and people were involved?

---

[41] The Bible calls this kind of change in direction "*repentance.*"

Being tired can cause many of us to be less vigilant to guard our boundaries. But, if we renew our minds when tired, *even before we are tempted*, we will strengthen and steady ourselves with God's Big T Truth personalized for the current situation:

"I can do ALL things through Christ Who strengthens me![42] Lord, I will make it through this day with my boundaries in tact. Even though I am tired, I will be vigilant today and depend on the strength you have promised me for this day. Eating when I am not hungry (or *over*eating), will likely cause me to feel more tired and lethargic. I commit my eating and my body afresh to You before I begin this day."

"Because I am so vulnerable, I won't do the grocery shopping today. I will wait until I am not as likely to buy everything in sight."

"Because I feel weaker today, I will call a Thin Within buddy to pray with me."

> **Each morning, we can prepare for the day ahead by wall-papering our minds with Truth.**

When we apply the Truth to our situations, we no longer perpetuate failure through self-condemnation. For instance, we can prepare in advance for our meeting with a difficult person who has previously agitated us, by renewing our minds *proactively*:

"Lord, you have called me to this work relationship. You have given me everything I need for life and godliness, including the ability to refuse to give in to overeating when I am nervous (agitated, intimidated, overwhelmed, scared, excited). Lord, I put my hand in yours and choose to walk with you through this day and glorify you in my eating, drinking, and whatever I do."[43]

LEARN: Prayerfully ponder the situation you described and consider what you can learn from the experience. How can you prepare for success and victory the next time? What does God want you to do so that you can walk forward in faith, confident of victory ahead?

---

[42] Philippians 4:13
[43] 2 Peter 1:3; 1 Corinthians 10:31

© 2019 Heidi Bylsma, www.renewedlifementoring.com. All rights reserved. Printed in the United States of America. No part of this book may be used or reproduced in any matter whatsoever without written permission.

Consider your upcoming week. Do you see a potentially stressful or challenging situation ahead? How will you prepare yourself to be victorious and to keep your eating boundaries? Be specific.

_____

_____

_____

_____

Today, if you break your boundaries, **LOOK**. Pause and evaluate what was going on. What can you **LEARN** about yourself, about God, about your body, food, and eating? What can you do to be victorious next time?

_____

_____

_____

_____

Respond

What has the Lord shown you today? How would He like you to respond?

_____

_____

_____

_____

_____

_____

_____

© 2019 Heidi Bylsma, www.renewedlifementoring.com All rights reserved. Printed in the United States of America. No part of this book may be used or reproduced in any matter whatsoever without written permission.

LESSON 10

Scripture

But the hour is coming, and is now here,
when the true worshipers will worship the Father in spirit and truth,
for the Father is seeking such people to worship him.

John 4:23 (ESV)

Praise Him! ~ PraiseFest

You belong to Jesus. You are *His*. That is who you are. God has called you out of darkness to praise Him![44] So, today, we will do precisely that!

Look at the lists you made in Lessons 2 and 8. Those pages contain your "God List" (so far) and you can continue to add to it any time you want. Now, using any part of your God List, we are going to praise our God and King. Here is how –

If your God List from Lesson 2 has these answers:

- His love is steadfast.
- He gives refuge in the shadow of His wings.
- He is faithful.

…you may have added things in the fourth column such as

- He wants me to believe He will protect me.
- He wants me to believe He nurtures me.

We can praise God using these attributes. So, if you were to "PraiseFest" these attributes, it might sound something like this:

> Lord, Your love is steadfast. It never moves or runs out. You are my refuge. I can run to You and You will nurture and protect me. You are faithful to me, no matter what. I praise You for Your faithfulness, Lord God.

For greater impact, you can expand on what each means to you personally:

---

[44] 1 Peter 2:9

> *Lord, when no one else is faithful, YOU are. Thank you that I can count on You, even when there is more month than money or when the next trial hits before I have come up for air from the previous challenge!*

"PraiseFesting" out loud is very helpful—at home doing chores, in the shower, in the car after dropping kids off at school or Day Care, or on the way to work. Giving God praise He is due will impact us *and* others in our families. Let them hear you praising Him!

When we are tempted to munch when we aren't hungry, "PraiseFesting" for five minutes redirects our attention. Often, when we think we are hungry, it is actually a hunger for God that needs to be satisfied. Feeding heart hunger with physical food won't meet the need. But when we praise our God, we get a sense of satisfaction and fulfillment that physical food can't touch. He fills our hearts with His Presence.[45] Try it and see!

When I exalt God, I demonstrate that I accept my place as His child. I declare: "Your will, God. Your way, Your desires for me..." instead of "**My** will. **My** way. **My** food." When I develop a practice of praising God, exalting Him for His character and how kind He is, I take my rightful place and am less likely to overeat. He is the potter and I am the clay. He is **King**.

> **Praise is saying to God what He is like and thanking Him for Who He is and what He does for people.**

Conduct your PraiseFest using your God Lists from Lessons 2 and 8. Once you have done so, mark this box. ☐ How much time did it take? _____

What are your thoughts and impressions about your PraiseFest?

_____
_____
_____
_____
_____
_____
_____

---

[45] Psalm 22:3 KJV

© 2019 Heidi Bylsma, www.renewedlifementoring.com All rights reserved. Printed in the United States of America. No part of this book may be used or reproduced in any matter whatsoever without written permission.

What emotions describe how you felt praising God? How do you feel now? (Circle any that apply.)

Amazed	Free	Satisfied	Glad	Joyful Light-Hearted
Bored	Greedy	Loved	Hopeful	Agitated
Certain	Comforted	Hungry	Protected	Thankful
Happy	Ashamed	Doubtful	Discouraged	Anxious
Refreshed	Safe	Warm	Touched	

What do you notice about how praising God affects your emotions?

_____

_____

_____

_____

More "Look and Learn"

In previous lessons, we asked you to begin to follow what Thin Within calls the Keys to Conscious Eating. Here they are again for quick reference:

1. Eat when your body is hungry.
2. Eat in a calm environment by reducing distractions.
3. Eat when sitting.
4. Eat when your body and mind are relaxed.
5. Eat and drink only the things that your body loves.
6. Pay attention only to your food while eating.
7. Eat slowly, savoring each bite.
8. Stop before your body is full.

© 2019 Heidi Bylsma, www.renewedlifementoring.com. All rights reserved. Printed in the United States of America. No part of this book may be used or reproduced in any matter whatsoever without written permission.

You have been working on Keys 1 and 8, or what we call in Thin Within, 0 to 5 eating. Additionally, you've selected foods you love (Key #5) and have been eating more slowly (Key #7). You selected another Key to work on in Lesson 6. Which Key have you been working on?

_____

_____

_____

How is it going?

_____

_____

_____

Today, please add another Key that you will work on. Which will it be?

_____

_____

_____

Respond

What has the Lord shown you today? How would He like you to respond?

_____

_____

_____

LESSON 11

Scripture

Everything is permissible for me, but not all things are beneficial.
Everything is permissible for me, but I will not be enslaved by anything...

1 Corinthians 6:12 (AMP)

Phase 2 - Developing Discernment

In the previous lessons, you were invited to enjoy the flavors and textures of any food. This is Phase 1 of Thin Within—the "Freedom Phase." *All things are permissible.* We can eat a modest portion of any food we choose if we are hungry. What are some foods you have been savoring for the past ten lessons?

_____

_____

_____

_____

How do you feel casting aside "good foods" and "bad foods" lists? What concerns do you have? What joys have you experienced?

_____

_____

_____

_____

On a scale of 1 to 10, how convinced are you that you can release extra weight and maintain your God-given size while selecting foods you enjoy?

1	2	3	4	5	6	7	8	9	10
Not at all				Possibly?					Definitely!

We will enjoy this pleasure our entire lives as we follow hunger and satisfaction cues. What an amazing gift! We will appreciate and embrace our freedom **now**, not just *to* eat foods we love, but also *from having to* eat those foods we love.

What food is hard for you to resist if it is available? It may seem to magnetically pull you closer. It calls your name from the freezer or desk drawer. Relentlessly. Each night. Or each day at 3pm. Or the moment the kids are in bed. Or when you walk past the break room. (We will talk in a future lesson about emotional attachments we may have to specific foods.)

We want to build our awareness throughout the rest of our time together.

Foods you select vary in their ability to energize and sustain you. Some do "just the trick" to fuel your body. Others may cause lethargy. God masterfully created your body! "Study" your body's responses to different foods eaten at 0. Let's start exercising godly discernment—Phase 2, is the Discernment Phase.

> **We will appreciate and embrace our freedom *now*… not just *to* eat foods we love, but also *from having to* eat those foods.**

Continue to walk in freedom from lists of "good" and "bad" foods that are designed by *others*. We even recommend eliminating terms like "junk food" and "healthy food." These tend to emotionally charge various foods.

Instead, start a running list in the space provided of the foods you enjoy, which are worth extra preparation or effort to get, **and** that consistently fuel your body well without negative consequences. Thin Within calls these "Whole Body Pleasers." Unlike lists from our dieting days, our Whole Body Pleaser lists will be as unique as our bodies are from one another! One person's Whole Body Pleaser might be a "Total Reject" for another. Note how your body reacts when you eat a particular food between 0 and 5. What works best for your body to eat for your first meal of the day? This may be the most important 0, establishing a tone for the whole day ahead. Add new foods to your list over time.

In the Discernment Phase, our goal becomes selecting Whole Body Pleasers more frequently, exercising our freedom *from having to* eat less beneficial foods. You might want to bookmark this page so you can keep updating your list.

<u>My Whole Body Pleasers</u>

_____

_____

_____

_____

Thin Within wisely reminds us of 1 Corinthians 6:12 that tells us all things are permissible, but not all are beneficial. Some foods—no matter how good they taste in the moment—may upset your stomach or add harmful chemicals to your body causing muscle and joint pain, while other foods give you energy and sustain you for quite a while. We can take note of foods that cause a negative response in our bodies or, when eaten first thing in the morning, cause us to feel lethargic within an hour or two. Thin Within calls these "Total Rejects." What are some of your Total Rejects?

<u>My Total Rejects</u>

_____

_____

_____

_____

Feast on the Word

What do Philippians 1:9-11 and Hebrews 5:14 say about discernment? How does this relate to you? Be as thorough as possible.

_____

_____

_____

_____

How do you think being more discerning when eating 0 to 5 will impact you emotionally, spiritually, and physically?

_____

_____

_____

_____

To Release Weight

Are you having victory with the Keys to Conscious Eating? Below, place a checkmark (✓) next to each key you feel relatively comfortable with.

Place an ✗ next to the keys you are working on that are the most challenging for you.

Place a star (★) next to any key you think might be helpful to start on next.

_____ 1. Eat when your body is hungry.

_____ 2. Eat in a calm environment by reducing distractions.

____ 3. Eat when sitting.

____ 4. Eat when your body and mind are relaxed.

____ 5. Eat and drink only the food that your body loves.

____ 6. Pay attention only to your food while eating. [46]

____ 7. Eat slowly, savoring each bite.

____ 8. Stop before your body is full.

What is working for you? What is challenging for you?

_____

_____

_____

_____

Today, as you discern your Total Rejects and Whole Body Pleasers, quiet your mind (Key 4)—even if in a noisy environment. Focus on the food as you eat, noting the textures and flavors when you take a bite (Key 6). Check in with your body, noting its response to the food eaten. Make observations throughout the day:

_____

_____

_____

_____

_____

_____

_____

_____

[46] Establish a rhythm when you are with other people so you can focus on your food and enjoy the company of others simultaneously.

© 2019 Heidi Bylsma, www.renewedlifementoring.com All rights reserved. Printed in the United States of America. No part of this book may be used or reproduced in any matter whatsoever without written permission.

Respond

What has the Lord shown you today? How would He like you to respond?

LESSON 12

Scripture

This is what the Sovereign Lord, the Holy One of Israel, says:
"In repentance and rest is your salvation,
in quietness and trust is your strength…"

Isaiah 30:15 (NIV)

In Lesson 11, we invited you to discern tastes, textures, and your body's responses to various food choices. You used your observations to begin your Whole Body Pleasers and Total Rejects lists. Continue to add to these lists today.

Feasting on God's Word

Look up these passages in your Bible and describe what you discover about God's invitation to His people:

Isaiah 55:2

_____

_____

Revelation 22:17

_____

_____

Isaiah 30:15

_____

_____

2 Corinthians 12:9-10

_____

_____

Hebrews 4:16

_____

_____

Jeremiah 6:16

_____

_____

> Optional:
>
> ** For extra credit ☺ and encouragement, add anything you learn about God and what He does for people from these verses to your **God List** (the list we began in lesson 2 about what God is like, what He does for people.
>
> *** For even *more* encouragement, use what you have added to enjoy another PraiseFest, praying your list of what God is like back to Him, exalting Him for Who He is and what He is like.

S.T.A.L.L. for Victory!

One creative Thin Within participant created the "S.T.A.L.L."[47] tool to help her to remember to evaluate whether she needs food and is truly physically hungry. We also love this tool for stopping *during* a meal to evaluate whether you still need more food.

S – Stop. First, we ***stop*** and ask the Lord what is drawing us to food. If physical need, our stomachs will often signal a clear 0. The stomach is located to the left of the center of our bodies behind and below where our ribs come together in our sternums (not in the abdomen). Stopping in this moment is an act of obedience, in which we tell the Lord, "I recognize that You would like to offer Your input about this!" (See Jeremiah 6:16).

T – Turn. Next, we ***turn*** away from the kitchen, the pantry, the drive-through, the plate, etc. Sometimes this is a physical turning away for just a moment. We take our affections off food, and focus our hearts, instead, on Jesus (1 Thessalonians 1:9).

A – Ask. We then ***ask*** the Lord what is going on. Is this desire to eat (or to keep eating) directed by my body's need for fuel? Is this physical hunger? Or is it heart or head hunger? What fuel might be best for my body in this moment? As we ask the Lord what is drawing us to food, we open ourselves to His way out of the temptation to break our boundaries (1 Corinthians 10:13).

L – Listen. A vital step, we then ***listen*** to what the Lord impresses upon our hearts. The Holy Spirit lives in hearts of those who profess Jesus as Lord. As we listen, we may not hear a voice audibly, but He will impress His answer on our hearts and minds or grant wisdom to know the right choice (1 Corinthians 2:14).

---

[47] We use this tool with her permission.

L – Learn and Love. We can *stop*, *turn*, *ask*, and even listen; but this second "L" is vital. We want to *learn* what God has for us in this place. We asked, he answered. We go a bit further and ask Him to show us how to **love** what He has impressed upon our hearts (Psalm 119:165). Whatever He tells us, we want to learn it and love and welcome it. His direction is what is best.

To Release Weight

Thin Within encourages us to have an:

Ideal Meal Experience

Today, plan for one special meal you will enjoy within the next few days. You will follow Thin Within's Keys to Conscious Eating. It may take some careful preparation, so have fun with this! It will be worth it!

> As we ask the Lord what is drawing us to food, we open ourselves to His way out of the temptation to break our boundaries.

Here they are again:

1. Eat when your body is hungry.
2. Eat in a calm environment by reducing distractions.
3. Eat when sitting.
4. Eat when your body and mind are relaxed.
5. Eat and drink only the things that your body loves.
6. Pay attention only to your food while eating.
7. Eat slowly, savoring each bite.
8. Stop before your body is full.

If today won't work, set a time for an "Ideal Meal" this week. For this exercise, select Whole Body Pleaser foods, a calm environment (consider getting a babysitter if you need to), no distractions, and the ideal ambience. You will slowly savor the food and relish your dining experience. Some participants set the table as if for an honored Guest and prayerfully invite Jesus to join them. Use this to worship Him for His provision, His presence, and His incredible creativity in available tastes and textures!

As you progress in your Thin Within journey, you can set up different "Ideal Meal Experiences." A sporting event done with all the keys to conscious eating, for instance. A holiday dinner with family and friends while practicing the keys. There is no end to the types of situations where you might want to have an "Ideal Meal Experience." Start with the simplest and challenge yourself as time goes on.

What day and time will you enjoy your meal?

© 2019 Heidi Bylsma, www.renewedlifementoring.com All rights reserved. Printed in the United States of America. No part of this book may be used or reproduced in any matter whatsoever without written permission.

Where will you eat your Ideal Meal?

What foods might you select?

Who will join you or will you be alone?

What do you need to do to enjoy this time in a quiet, stress-free manner, preferably uninterrupted?

What other special arrangements do you need to make in order for this to happen?

What do you think about this exercise?

Check this box when you have made your plan. ☐

    Remember to apply all the Keys to Conscious Eating during this meal and welcome God to your table. Some have found it very helpful to use this exercise whenever they need to "calibrate" – or remember what it is like to be intentional and present in the moment with their food, enjoying the Lord and His bounty within the boundaries of physical hunger and satisfaction. We will follow up with you about this in Lesson 13.

Respond

What has the Lord shown you today? How would He like you to respond?

LESSON 13

Scripture

> *For though we walk in the flesh,*
> *we are not waging war according to the flesh.*
> *For the weapons of our warfare are not of the flesh*
> *but have divine power to destroy strongholds.*
> *We destroy arguments and every lofty opinion*
> *raised against the knowledge of God,*
> *and take every thought captive to obey Christ...*
>
> 2 Corinthians 10:3-5 (ESV)

Getting to Know Our God, Part 1

How much time have I spent thinking about "the food *I* want to eat, the struggles *I* have, the size *I* want to be?" Diets often focus our attention on a worldly mindset. The best way to get our eyes off ourselves is to set our eyes on our amazing God and King. Praising God fills our hearts and minds with *Him*. As we do this, heart hunger and head hunger are less likely to lead us to eat food outside of physical hunger and satisfaction. We experience a "fullness" physical food can't give us, but one God promises is ours in Christ.[48]

> **We are not transformed by following our boundaries; we are transformed by the *renewing of our minds*.**

During the next four lessons, we will plunge the depths of God's character. We will meet the living God in the pages of His powerful Word. If you haven't started a separate God List yet, you might want to now. Again, we are not transformed by following our eating boundaries; we are transformed by the *renewing of our minds* (Romans 12:2). In order to *be* different, we need to *think* differently—about ourselves, about food, about our bodies and most importantly, about God!

---

[48] Colossians 2:9

A Personal Word…

This came home to me when, in 2006, I asked God why I felt stuck in Romans 7…the good I wanted to do was not what I did, but the very thing I didn't want to do is what I did. I had known about Thin Within and collaborated with the Hallidays on the book, *Thin Within,* and workbooks. I shared my testimony in the videos that went out to in-person group leaders—even before it was a weight-loss testimony.

Not only was I frustrated, but my heart was aching…and my ankles and knees, too, as I struggled with obesity. I asked God what was hindering me from doing what I knew would bring peace and the answer was clear, "You resent Me." As I spent time in His Word and prayer, I realized that I did, indeed, resent God. I felt like He expected too much of me in a permanent situation that I felt ill-equipped to handle. He was holding out on me…or so my errant thinking went.

> **As I spent time in His Word and prayer, I realized that I did, indeed, resent God.**

God invited me to come to the Word to learn from Him *about* Him. I had been focusing so much on my struggles that I had failed to keep my eyes on what He is truly like. That is how the God List was born. As I began to use the God List to be reminded of the fullness and awesomeness of God's character, as I used it to praise and exalt Him, life became less about *my* will, *my* way, *my* struggle, *my* weight, and more about God's will, God's way, God's goodness.

I hope that you find the continued process of reviewing the truth about the Lord an encouragement, providing the breakthrough that you hope for.

What are your thoughts as you begin this exploration? Use the provided space to record a prayer that the Lord will reveal Himself to you during today's study.

_____

_____

_____

_____

Please look up the verses on the following pages. Beside each, write down what God is like, what He does for people, and what He wants you to believeAdd these to your comprehensive God List as well.

Verse To Look Up	What God is Like	What He Does for People	What He Wants me to Believe
Psalm 102:12-13			
Romans 8:28			
Exodus 34:6-7			
Psalm 25:8			
Psalm 145:17			
Romans 3:23-24			
Ephesians 4:7			

Hebrews 4:16			
Psalm 99:2-3			
Isaiah 6:3			
Revelation 4:8			

To Release Weight

Getting to know our God more intimately is a wonderful benefit of this journey. The truth of Who He is will make a practical difference in our lives and in our challenges with eating. Whenever my eating is "off," it is a barometer for me telling me that I haven't been surrendering to God's sovereignty or spending time praising Him. Sometimes, this is rooted in lies that I believe without even realizing it.

In the column on the left in the following chart, jot down statements you know are lies or little t truths. These include beliefs you've held for the past twelve lessons. In the right-hand column, write down a corresponding Truth about God—the Big T Truth—that trumps the lie or little t truth you listed.

Lie or "little t truth"	"Big T Truth"
God did this *to* me.	God did this *for* me. He intends it for my growth and good.
I am on my own to deal with challenges in life.	God invites me to come to him for mercy, grace, and help.

For added impact, put a single line through each lie or little t truth. Now, asterisk, star, *and* circle the Big T Truth. Get out your Truth Cards/Truth List and write each statement from the right hand column on a new card. *When you have done that, check this box.* ☐

Whenever you are tempted to break your boundaries today, try a couple of the tools we have introduced so far. From lesson 12, you can use the S.T.A.L.L. tool for a moment. Spend 5 minutes going through the Truth Cards or reading through your Truth List you created. You can even make a "bargain" with yourself… *"After I have renewed my mind for five minutes, I can eat the _(insert favorite morsel here)_ if I still want it."* Once we have renewed our minds, we typically don't *want* to eat outside our boundaries after all! Jot down your observations once you have done this today:

_____

_____

_____

Have you planned your Ideal Meal Experience yet?   Yes   No

If not, when do you plan to do so? _____

In Lesson 14, we will ask you to write about your Ideal Meal Experience. If you have already completed this assignment from Lesson 12, you are welcome to turn to Lesson 14 and respond to the questions about your meal.

© 2019 Heidi Bylsma, www.renewedlifementoring.com. All rights reserved. Printed in the United States of America. No part of this book may be used or reproduced in any matter whatsoever without written permission.

Respond

What has the Lord shown you today? How would He like you to respond?

LESSON 14

Scripture

"Great and amazing are your deeds, O Lord God the Almighty!
Just and true are your ways, O King of the nations!
Who will not fear, O Lord, and glorify your name?
For you alone are holy.
All nations will come and worship you,
for your righteous acts have been revealed."

Revelation 15:3b-4 (ESV)

Getting to Know Our God, Part 2

Sometimes we don't even know our hearts are resentful toward God. After all, good Christian folks don't *feel* that way. Or do they? Through any of life's circumstances—a miscarriage, broken marriage, church split, loss of a job, medical test results—if we don't keep our eyes riveted on our God and His compassion and love, we will start running from the pain or stuffing it. We often turn to food in these moments. Problem is, looking to food for comfort, means we aren't likely to experience the comfort that God has in mind for us. The pain is there, lurking beneath the surface and likely to jump out at us at the most inopportune moment.

Blessed be the God and Father of our Lord Jesus Christ, the Father of mercies and God of all comfort, who comforts us in all our affliction, so that we may be able to comfort those who are in any affliction, with the comfort with which we ourselves are comforted by God.

2 Corinthians 1:3-4

Let's continue the process we began and broaden our knowledge of the amazing God we worship. Take some time today to add to your God List. Invite God into this study time; ask Him to show you how praising and exalting Him will transform your heart. Think about the impact getting to know God more intimately might have on your decisions to glorify Him with your eating and drinking (1 Corinthians 10:31).

> **If we don't keep our eyes riveted on our God and His compassion and love, we will start running from the pain or stuffing it.**

Please look up the following verses. Next to each, write down what God is like, what He does for people, and what He wants you to believe as a result. Add these to your comprehensive God List or Truth Cards/List as well.

Verse To Look Up	What God is Like / What He Does for People	What He Wants me to Believe
Acts 17:27-28		
Malachi 3:6		
Nehemiah 9:32a		
John 3:16		
Romans 5:4-5		
Romans 5:8		
Romans 8:35, 39		
1 John 4:16		
Ephesians 2:4		
Titus 3:5		

What do you love the most about God from our study today? Why?

___

As you did in Lesson 13, take five minutes to have a PraiseFest, exalting and thanking God for the truth of Who He is and the attributes of His character you gleaned from today's study. Journal here about your time of praising God:

___

Did you skip the above PraiseFest opportunity? ☺   Yes ☐   No ☐

Why?

___

Today, if food comes to mind when you're not hungry, turn to your God List or other exercises you've completed in this workbook. Use them to have a PraiseFest—out loud if you can—directing your attention away from the food. Record what happens when you do on the following page. The first entry is an example to guide you.

Time of Temptation	Nature of Temptation	What I Did to Redirect My Attention	Outcome
2:00 pm Saturday at home	Wanted a second helping of lunch even though I was physically satisfied.	Used my God List for 5 minutes; praised and exalted God for Who He is.	Got my mind off the food and back on God. Moved on in my day. Victory!

To Release Weight

During the last few lessons we have encouraged you to prayerfully use discernment in selecting your foods, noting how each food eaten between the boundaries of 0 and 5 causes you to feel. Have you added to your list of Whole Body Pleasers from Lesson 11? Have you noticed which foods are Total Rejects for you? These lists include drinks as well as foods. As you continue your journey, both lists will grow and change. In time, some foods you had on your Total Rejects List might actually make it to your Whole Body Pleasers List. The opposite may also be true!

Another category of foods we will develop discernment about is what Thin Within calls "Taste Bud Teasers." These are foods you typically *don't* think about or plan for ahead of time but may appeal to you if left open and available on the kitchen counter or if you catch the scent of it baking. For example, the sweet smell of cinnamon breakfast rolls in the oven may seem difficult to resist or you may mindlessly grab a handful of pretzels when you walk through the kitchen. Once we start eating these Taste Bud Teasers we tend to keep munching on them without giving a thought to the Keys to Conscious Eating. These foods may be a temporary delight to our taste buds, but they don't usually do much to *satisfy* physical hunger.

> **God has placed a God-shaped void in each one of us we call "heart hunger." If we don't fill that hole with Him, we may reach for food or other temporary, ineffective "fixes."**

Taste Bud Teasers are often what we grab when we eat to stuff down our emotions. God has placed a God-shaped void in each one of us we call "heart hunger." If we don't fill that hole with Him, we may reach for food or other temporary, ineffective "fixes."

Sometimes we want to crunch on something due to stress or agitation of some sort. But the truth is, once we have eaten Taste Bud Teasers we feel like we still need "real food" even if we aren't hungry!

What are your Taste Bud Teasers? You may have ideas come to you right away or you may have to use discernment throughout the day to come up with a list. Keep a record of your Taste Bud Teasers in the space provided and continue to add to your Total Rejects and Whole Body Pleasers lists in Lesson 11.

My Taste Bud Teasers

_____

_____

_____

_____

Ideal Meal Experience Reflection[49]

In Lesson 12, we asked you to plan an eating occasion where you could practice all the Keys to Conscious Eating. How did you feel about this experience? What did you learn about eating? About yourself? About God? What keys did you have success with? What keys were the most challenging for you? Record your thoughts here:

_____

_____

_____

_____

_____

---

[49] If it seems too overwhelming to try to do this activity applying ALL of the Keys to Conscious Eating, please select 2 or 3 of the keys to focus on, instead.

© 2019 Heidi Bylsma, www.renewedlifementoring.com. All rights reserved. Printed in the United States of America. No part of this book may be used or reproduced in any matter whatsoever without written permission.

Respond

What has the Lord shown you today? How would He like you to respond?

LESSON 15

Scripture

For God gave us a spirit not of fear
but of power and love and self-control.

2 Timothy 1:7 (ESV)

For God so loved the world, that he gave his only Son,
that whoever believes in him
should not perish but have eternal life.

John 3:16 (ESV)

Getting to Know Our God, Part 3

We've only just begun to unearth the vastness of the treasure that is our God and all that he is and does for people. Let's ask the Lord to deepen and widen our view of Who He is. As we develop our understanding of how big God is, our faith grows, and we are able to trust Him with more of our lives. This includes glorifying Him with our eating and drinking (1 Corinthians 10:31).

Look up the following verses. Next to each, as before, write down what God is like, what He does for people, and what He wants you to believe. Add these to your comprehensive God List. Isn't it wonderful that God lovingly reveals Himself to us through His living Word?

Verse To Look Up	What God is Like	What He Does for People	What He Wants me to Believe
Hebrews 1:3			
Jeremiah 32:17			
Matthew 19:26			

Now, enjoy a five to ten-minute PraiseFest. Then, write thoughts about your study, God List, and PraiseFest. How is your relationship with your loving Savior deepening?

_____

_____

_____

_____

The past three lessons have painted a powerful picture of God's Big T Truth. As God has revealed to you more of what He is like and what He does for people, have you also discovered some lies or little t truths you have believed? These stumbling blocks are removed as we take our thoughts and line them up with God's Big T Truth. On the lines provided, write any lies or little t truths God has brought to light in your life. Write down a corresponding Big T Truth that refutes each.

Lie or little t truth	**Big T Truth to refute it**

To Release Weight

We encourage you to tread a path not often traveled in this world. We will present our hearts and minds to God to be transformed. We do this rather than calling on our own self-effort to lose weight and get fit. Attaching blame to food and eating only things on a "good food list" is not the answer; we are learning how to renew our minds with Big T Truths from Scripture. You may now wonder, what place activity has in *Fresh Wind, Fresh Desire*.

Let's first take a look at what we do ***not*** teach about exercise. FWFD does NOT encourage:

- Avoiding exercise
- Using exercise as a means to lose weight
- Exercising **in**appropriately for your body
- The "no pain, no gain" mentality

- Using exercise as a reason to eat more

Psalm 115:3			
Job 11:7-9			
Jeremiah 23:23-24			
Psalm 139:7-10			
Psalm 90:1-2			
Psalm 147:5			
Romans 11:33			

- Exercising in order to burn off food you have already eaten

FWFD DOES encourage us to:

- Evaluate our bodies' need for exercise and how much.
    - When your body needs exercise, we liken that to a "0" just like we do when our bodies need food. Our bodies need to move each day. This can include doing chores, such as cutting the grass and vacuuming, recreational exercise like tennis or golf, or a delightful swim at the local YMCA.
- Select activities we enjoy… just like we choose foods we enjoy.
    - Jot below which movement activities energize and delight you:

_____

_____

© 2019 Heidi Bylsma, www.renewedlifementoring.com. All rights reserved. Printed in the United States of America. No part of this book may be used or reproduced in any matter whatsoever without written permission.

- Renew our minds about exercise if we have either avoided or overused it in the past.

    - What lies or little t truths do you believe about exercise? Ask the Lord to show you *His* will for *you* personally regarding exercise.

- Stop exercising when our bodies have had enough.

    - When we eat 0 to 5, we stop at the point where the body is satisfied. In the same way, unless you are an endurance athlete training for an event, stop exercising when your body has had just enough. More is not necessarily better.

- Participate in activity appropriate for our physical condition.

    - Many things can affect our ability to exercise at varying degrees. Whether you are able to do chores around the house, walk your dog around the block, hike a trail in the mountains, run a marathon, or move your arms while staying seated, God will show you the activity (and how much of it) that is best for you.

- Use Christian music to make movement of *any* kind a worship experience!

When we are active, we continue to eat according to cues of hunger and satisfaction. I enjoy hiking in the mountains with my dog. Some days I enjoy a longer, more strenuous hike and other days a short walk with a dip in the river is just enough. If I know ahead of time that I will hike five miles at 8am the next morning, I plan my hunger by adjusting what and when I eat the night before. This way. I wake up hungry and enjoy a small breakfast before I leave. Packing Whole Body Pleasers in my backpack, I am prepared if I get hungry before the end of the hike. Usually a few bites is all I need.

What lies or little t truths do you believe about exercise?

_____

_____

_____

_____

Take a moment to pray, asking God what *His* view of moving your body is. If it helps, imagine Jesus is sitting next to you and discussing this with you. He loves you and is passionate for your joy! You can write Big T Truths for each little t truth you recorded in the previous question.

_____

_____

_____

_____

Add any Big T Truths to your Truth Cards/God List. *Check this box when done.* ☐

If you don't know what activities you might enjoy, here are some ideas to jumpstart your imagination:

- Plant and keep up a garden.
- Dance in your living room to your favorite music.
- Use workout DVDs and enjoy a variety of exercise at home.
- Go Geocaching and participate in a treasure hunt. (See **http://www.geocaching.com** to learn more.)
- Take a bicycle ride with a friend.
- Create an indoor obstacle course with your kids or grandkids on a rainy day.
- Play an active game like charades with your family.
- Try something new like stand-up paddle boarding. It's a blast!
- Test out an exercise subscription service. These services are social media-like communities, but they stream exercise classes live! (Just don't get sucked back into the diet mentality that sometimes accompanies these services.)

Respond

What has the Lord shown you today? How would He like you to respond?

_____

_____

_____

_____

_____

_____

LESSON 16

Scripture

Trust in the Lord and do good;
dwell in the land and enjoy safe pasture.
Take delight in the Lord,
and he will give you the desires of your heart.
Commit your way to the Lord;
trust in him and he will do this:
He will make your righteous reward shine like the dawn,
your vindication like the noonday sun.

Psalm 37:3-6 (NIV)

Getting to Know Our God, Part 4

Let's further expand our understanding of our God. These four lessons of study are intense; but we believe the result will be a larger, more comprehensive view of God, deeper intimacy with Him, and the ability to trust Him with more of our needs than ever before. Your personal God List will encourage you any time you need it. Use it to have a PraiseFest whenever you need to be reminded of how great our God is in comparison to your challenges!

> **Sometimes, the best gift we can give ourselves is to take our focus off our weight.**

Please take a moment to invite God into this study time.

_____
_____
_____
_____

Look up the verses on the following pages. What is God like, what does He do for people, and what does He want you to believe? Add these to your comprehensive God List.

Verse To Look Up	What God is Like / What He Does for People	What He Wants me to Believe
Psalm 19:7		
Isaiah 5:16		
Isaiah 45:21		
John 1:1-5		
Colossians 1:15-17		
Matthew 10:29		
Daniel 2:21-22		

© 2019 Heidi Bylsma, www.renewedlifementoring.com. All rights reserved. Printed in the United States of America. No part of this book may be used or reproduced in any matter whatsoever without written permission.

Isaiah 55:8-9		
Isaiah 57:15		

Lift our mighty God and King up in praise, using what you have found in His Word today. Record your thoughts about your PraiseFest here:

___

___

___

___

What lies or little t truths have you become aware of today? What Big T Truths will you replace them with?

___

___

Add any new Big T Truths to your Truth Cards and then check this box: ☐

To Release Weight

Sometimes, the best gift we can give ourselves is to take our focus *off* our weight. For the past four lessons, we have studied a lot of Scripture offering a beautiful description of what God is like and His kindness to people. We hope, in doing so, you are spurred into a more intimate relationship with our amazing God—He longs for closeness with you, His chosen child.

> **Let's be proactive to cut off temptation *before* it hits. It might take just five or ten minutes, but change the direction of the rest of our day!**

Only *He* can satisfy us. He provides physical food to meet our physical hunger, but going to physical food when we have a God-shaped hole in our hearts will not only *not* fill our emptiness, it will make us feel worse. God wants to flood the God-shaped void with *His* Holy Spirit, but He will wait for an invitation.[50] In praising God for Who the Scriptures reveal Him to be, we may be more likely to turn to Him instead of all the counterfeits that beckon us.

As we move our focus off food and ourselves and place it on God, life becomes about *His* will, *His* way, *His* plan for my eating (and life!), and *His* intended size for me instead of *my* will and *my* way. As I exalt God, I don't exalt myself like I do when I insist on eating outside the boundaries God has given me. When I draw closer in intimacy to God, I break my eating boundaries and grab for excess food *much* less frequently. My renewed mind informs me instantly that a marvelous God has purchased me with the blood of Jesus. He has paid an exorbitant price for me to belong to Him! I am only a steward of this remarkable body, fearfully and wonderfully made.

Many of us struggle with overeating during the late afternoon or evening hours. If you can identify the reason this time is especially challenging, you can prayerfully "dismantle" the situation and apply God's Big T Truth to it. One strategy to overcome this tendency is to renew our minds just before the time of day when we are most tempted to break our boundaries. We can use our Truth Cards, add to our God Lists, or have a PraiseFest. Let's be proactive to cut off temptation *before* it hits. It might take five or ten minutes, but change the direction of the rest of our day!

Record here what you did and how it made a difference for you today.

_____

_____

_____

_____

Respond

What has the Lord shown you today? How would He like you to respond?

_____

_____

_____

_____

_____

_____

_____

---

[50] 2 Corinthians 3:17

LESSON 17

Scripture

Know that the Lord, he is God!
It is he who made us, and we are his;
we are his people, and the sheep of his pasture.

Psalm 100:3 (NIV)

The Lord is my shepherd; I shall not want.

Psalm 23:1 (ESV)

He will tend his flock like a shepherd;
he will gather the lambs in his arms;
he will carry them in his bosom,
and gently lead those that are with young.

Isaiah 40:11 (ESV)

How Much is Enough?

It is God's great and glorious nature to give. He supplies all we need, day in and day out.

But do you ever feel like you just can't get enough? Precious time spent with a friend or family member? Money? Vacations? Breaks from trials?

At a buffet lunch, church potluck, or a Super Bowl party, we load up our plates as if we can't get enough food. What foods land on your plate in situations like this? Often, it will be foods on our Taste Bud Teaser List. What are some examples of eating occasions when you have said to yourself: "Just a bit more" or "One more piece"?

_____

_____

_____

What are some "little t truths" or downright lies that might have fueled your choice to overeat during those moments?

_____

_____

_____

_____

Right now, prayerfully dismantle what precedes the choice made to overeat in these situations. Is it anticipating the event hours before—even the day prior? Do you plan for *obedience*? Or are your plans less virtuous? What is going on during the moments when you give in to the temptation to overeat?

_____

_____

_____

_____

_____

If you aren't hungry and grab for food regardless of what your body needs, breaking your eating boundaries, how much will be enough to satisfy you?

_____

_____

_____

_____

_____

As we ask God to show us His "Big T Truth," we know that He will be faithful to shine His light on the lies and "little t truths" we want to eliminate from our lives. First, let us be clear about this:

> God has demonstrated His love for us **even while we were yet rebellious people**—before we ever got our "acts" together—**Christ died** for us (Romans 5:8). Ephesians 1:5 tells us that before the foundation of the

> world, he chose us to be holy and blameless in his sight and that, in love, he predestined us to be adopted as His children. Without you or me picking up a bible, giving an offering, or doing a good deed, **God chose us.**
>
> But that isn't all. In John 3:17, God tells us that he didn't send His Son into the world to condemn the world, but to save the world. In Romans 8:1 we are told there is *no* condemnation for those who are in Christ Jesus.

Look at the text in the box above. Underline the words and phrases that describe what the Lord of the Universe sees in you or has done for you. *Mark this box when you have done that.* ☐

With glorious awareness that God doesn't condemn us, let's embrace an eternal perspective, tilling and cultivating the soil of our hearts, opening to the fresh wind of the Holy Spirit to continue to stir a fresh desire to hold nothing back from Him. If you begin to feel a sense of condemnation, please know that it isn't because the Lord is condemning you! He *is not!* The Holy Spirit may bring *conviction* as we work through today's lesson. Conviction is a very *specific* sense of what we need to change. His divine power gives us *everything*—not just *some*—of what we need, for life and godliness (2 Peter 1:3).

> **With glorious awareness that God doesn't condemn us, let's embrace an eternal perspective.**

The Enemy of our souls, on the other hand, brings a general sense of condemnation—a feeling of worthlessness that says "I AM a failure. I AM condemned." These are LIES. What is God's Big T Truth? Remember that the overarching purposes of God are always for our good and His glory! He does *not* condemn us. We can't "let God down" because we aren't *holding him up* in the first place!

Keeping these Big T Truths in mind, let's dare to look at:

Greed

We give our time and our money to serve our families, friends and others in need. But do we allow our taste buds to rule us on occasion and over-ride our good reason and tender heart for God? Why? Often it may be because lurking *very* deep beneath the surface are more lies and little t truths influencing us. This is why we must renew our minds! Renewing our minds is one of the best life-long commitments we can make.

Wanting more than we need just because we want it...or because we like it...or because everyone else is doing it...may be rooted in an attitude of entitlement and not in God's Big T Truth. What *is* true? What is true is that Romans 3:23 and Romans 6:23 make it clear that we all fall short of the glory of God and deserve *death*. But rather than condemn us to hell—*because of the cross of Christ*—God chose to give us, His favored children, every spiritual blessing! He has adopted us. We are *His* (1 John 2:1-2)!

> **Our God is *crazy* about you. He delights over you.**

Our God is *crazy* about you. He delights over you. He quiets you with His love (Zephaniah 3:17). He is enthralled by your beauty (Psalm 45:11). He has invited you to be His. This is God's Truth for you!

Renewing our minds with God's Truth, we think His thoughts after Him. We ask His view of people, situations, and concerns, adopting what He impresses upon our hearts—His eternal perspective. Often it comes from applying the Truth found in Scripture specifically to our situations, answering a question like: "If Jesus was sitting beside me, what would *He* tell me is true in this moment?" This goes beyond the typical prayer time and bible reading that we assume is a part of growing, maturing believers in the Lord Jesus Christ. This process of renewing our minds is even *more* work than that!

> **If Jesus was sitting beside me, what would *He* tell me is true in this moment?**

It is right and good and God-honoring to ask Him what His view is on the subject of over-eating. We, at Thin Within, get asked all the time if eating one bite past a 5 is a sin. Romans 14 says that whatever we do that is not done in faith is sin. If you can't eat the next bite in faith, then perhaps it *is* sin (Romans 14:23). No one can determine this for another. When the Holy Spirit brings conviction, let's respond lovingly to His direction. He will never *condemn*.

Greed and entitlement affect how much we choose to eat. If we were without a shred of greed or an ounce of an attitude of entitlement, would we overeat? We submit to you that it isn't likely. Even motivators like stress, boredom, seeking satisfaction have an underlying lie fueling them. What do you think that lie might be?

_____

_____

_____

_____

Do we believe a subtle lie that we are entitled to what Barb Raveling[51] calls in her books and Bible studies "the Good Life?" In "the Good Life" everything should be easy, fun and feel good. If things aren't easy, fun and feel good, we'll turn to food because we are entitled to feel better and have fun. Even if it is more food than I need, I act as though I am entitled to it. Can you identify? How so?

> **We are blessedly free from condemnation.**

_____

_____

_____

_____

---

[51] Barb Raveling, while not a Thin Within participant, is a master of mind renewal strategies and has been the source of much inspiration as we have developed this curriculum.

© 2019 Heidi Bylsma, www.renewedlifementoring.com. All rights reserved. Printed in the United States of America. No part of this book may be used or reproduced in any matter whatsoever without written permission.

How does this connect to *greed?*

_____

_____

_____

_____

We want to have *God's* view of entitlement and greed, thinking *God's* thoughts after Him. Colossians 3:5 tells us what He says:

> *Put to death, therefore, whatever belongs to your earthly nature:*
> *sexual immorality, impurity, lust, evil desires and* **greed,**
> **which is idolatry** *(NIV).*

Idolatry!? Yes. An attitude of entitlement is typically rooted in greed, which Scripture says is idolatry! Thankfully, we are blessedly **free from condemnation** as we receive this truth with open hearts. The question is, what do we do with this Truth?

Make no mistake--we *swim* in grace, but we know that grace isn't an excuse to do whatever we want. In fact, the Holy Spirit is in us to enable us to make good, God-honoring choices. This is grace! We simply cannot ignore His leadership. We must invite God to show us His thoughts.[52] Only this way can we truly think His thoughts after Him:

> *For the grace of God has appeared, bringing salvation for all people,*
> *training us to renounce ungodliness and worldly passions,*
> *and to live self-controlled, upright, and godly lives in the present age...*
>
> Titus 2:11-12

In addition to the incredible gift of salvation, what does grace train us to do?

_____

_____

_____

What does our eating have to do with ungodliness, worldly passions or self-control?

_____

_____

_____

---

[52] 1 Corinthians 2:16

To Release Weight

Today, continue to practice all of the Keys to Conscious Eating. Also, serve yourself two-thirds to half as much food as you would have before beginning going through this workbook or starting Thin Within. Eat half as much twice as slowly and you will get as much enjoyment out of savoring a smaller portion in the same amount of time. Try this at least once each day for the next week, if not for each meal.

What can you add to your Truth Cards about what you believe about grace? About greed? About the Holy Spirit's Presence in your life?

_____

_____

_____

_____

When you have added these truths to your Truth Cards or Truth List, make a check mark here: ☐

Sometime today for 10 minutes review the Truth Cards or Truth List you have created so far. Reading them out loud is especially effective. *When you have done that, mark this box.* ☐

Respond

What has the Lord shown you today? How would He like you to respond?

_____

_____

_____

_____

_____

_____

_____

_____

© 2019 Heidi Bylsma, www.renewedlifementoring.com. All rights reserved. Printed in the United States of America. No part of this book may be used or reproduced in any matter whatsoever without written permission.

LESSON 18

Scripture

*Be sober-minded; be watchful.
Your adversary the devil prowls around
like a roaring lion, seeking someone to devour.*

1 Peter 5:8 (ESV)

*God made him who had no sin to be sin for us,
so that in him we might become
the righteousness of God.*

2 Corinthians 5:21 (NIV)

Guilt and Shame – Let's Get Rid Of It!

In Lesson 17, we saw that the Holy Spirit convicts us lovingly and specifically. He sheds light on precise behaviors that He wants us to adjust so that we might honor Him and respect the body that He has given us to steward. We relish the wonderful fact that *our bodies are not our own but were purchased by Jesus' blood and are the temple of the Holy Spirit*. We belong to Him! The enemy of our souls wants you and I to feel a general sense of condemnation, failure, guilt and shame. In fact, if he can get us to feel condemnation and guilt—if he can get us to consider ourselves failures or inadequate Christians—then he has undercut the very identity that Jesus died to provide us (please review Lesson 9).[53]

> **Renewing our minds will actually change our desires.**

We will act according to what we believe is true. Guilt and condemnation cause shame, which leads us to act in a way that perpetuates more guilt and condemnation, leading to yet more shame and more of the same or similar behavior that causes us to feel guilt and condemnation! The cycle looks like the figure to the right.

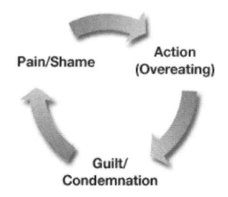

---

[53] 1 Corinthians 6:19-20, 1Peter 5:8, John 1:12

Unless we do something to stop this powerful cycle, we may keep the cycle going for years! Can you identify with the pain/shame cycle? How so? Please describe.

___

___

___

___

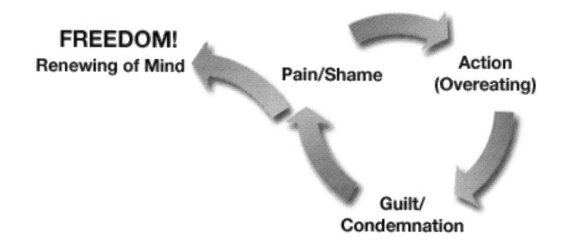

The struggle is even more challenging when we act entitled or greedy. It hinders our willingness to break free. We may lack *desire*. Renewing our minds will actually change our desires. Let's not leave this to chance! As our desires change, our behaviors will as well. We actually will *want* to act differently![54] Renewing our minds is a way to jump out of this cycle into freedom!

Take a moment right now to renew your mind with truth from your cards or lists. *Check the box when you have done that.* ☐

Without time and effort given to renew our minds, lasting change can't occur. But if we renew our minds daily, when we grab food out of habit, or to satisfy heart hunger, our renewed minds will engage with instruction and resolve—even **cause** us to

> **But if we renew our minds daily, when we grab food out of habit, or to satisfy heart hunger, our renewed minds will engage with instruction and resolve—even cause us to "want to" do the right thing!**

---

[54] Romans 12:2, Psalm 145:16

© 2019 Heidi Bylsma, www.renewedlifementoring.com. All rights reserved. Printed in the United States of America. No part of this book may be used or reproduced in any matter whatsoever without written permission.

"want to" do the right thing!55 We will *want to* say "No!" to the sensual indulgence that previously mastered us and say "Yes" to the godly choice.

Make It Personal

What are ways in which shame and guilt have affected your eating and your view of your body?

_____

_____

_____

_____

Which do you feel like you want more? To eat what you want in the amounts you want? Or to break free from a pain/shame cycle? Explain.

_____

_____

_____

_____

What will you give up to break free?

_____

_____

_____

_____

What do you plan to do to break free and when will you do that? Please be specific.

_____

_____

_____

_____

---

55 Titus 2:12

What Big T truths are in your previous answers?

_____
_____
_____
_____

In three months, what benefits will you experience if you take the actions that you wrote above, become free of the guilt-shame cycle, renew your mind daily, and start or continue to follow your eating boundaries?

_____
_____
_____
_____

What Big T truth is in your previous answer?

_____
_____
_____
_____

What consequences come from eating out of a sense of entitlement or greed?

_____
_____
_____
_____

What Big T truth is in your previous answer?

_____
_____
_____
_____

Is it worth what it will take to break free and live free?

_____

_____

_____

_____

Using the answers to "What Big T truth is in my previous answer?" create new truths for your cards or Truth List. *Mark this box when you have done so.* ☐

Review your truths for five minutes sometime today. *Mark this box when you have done so.* ☐

To Release Weight

God calls us to "abide in Him," to walk closely with Him, to breathe in His presence, to submit to Him in all things. He longs for deeper intimacy with us, lovingly drawing us in to a continual conversation with His Spirit. God invites us to deal with our food, eating and body issues and to eat within the boundaries of physical hunger and satisfaction. But what does it all look like practically?[56]

"Isn't breakfast the most important meal of the day?"

"But what if I'm not hungry for my lunch at my favorite restaurant?"

"I was famished at the grocery store the other day and bought everything in sight. What should I have done?"

"Shouldn't I eat three 'square' meals a day to get the nutrition I need?"

What questions do you have about the practical aspects of eating according to your body's signals of hunger and satisfaction?

_____

_____

_____

_____

_____

---

[56] John 15:4, Hebrews 10:22, Psalm 74:17

© 2019 Heidi Bylsma, www.renewedlifementoring.com All rights reserved. Printed in the United States of America. No part of this book may be used or reproduced in any matter whatsoever without written permission.

> **God calls us to "abide in Him," to walk closely with Him, to breathe in His presence, to submit to Him in all things. He longs for deeper intimacy with us, lovingly drawing us into a continual conversation with His Spirit.**

How can you get an answer to these questions? Be specific about what you will so and when. Consider reading *Thin Within*, getting involved in an online community, brainstorming with a like-minded friend.

God is doing a new thing. He calls us to see our bodies, our food and our eating in a new way. Let's continue to let go of the old rules and routines. Experiment with food and your eating in ways you may not have dared before. Let's look at how you can actually *plan* for your 0 to 5 eating in another practical way.[57]

> **God is doing a new thing. He calls us to see our bodies, our food and our eating in a new way.**

Practical Tip #1: We don't always know when we will be physically hungry. How do we balance this fact with our conviction not to eat outside of our God-given boundaries? A simple solution is to carry nuts, a nutrition bar, trail mix, or peanut M&Ms in your purse or backpack. A bit is all that is needed to keep you going strong through the meeting at work or a doctor's visit. These are typically discreet as well, so that even in the middle of church if your stomach signals that it is empty, you are able to quell the tide of hunger.

What food can you pack with you today (or tomorrow) so that you are equipped should you get hungry before you have a chance to sit down to a meal?

---

[57] Isaiah 43:19

Practical Tip #2a: To plan for a meal at a favorite restaurant at a specific time, you can strategize to land on empty by eating a smaller portion during the preceding meal. This is completely acceptable and often necessary! Extend grace to yourself as you learn this. It takes practice like riding a bike. At first, it will require focus, but, with observation and correction, over time, you will do it "naturally." You will find different foods "hold" you differently and in various amounts.

Practical Tip #2b: When you plan to eat within your boundaries, you prepare for a successful day. Take a few minutes each morning to look ahead at your day. What will your schedule be? Will you be eating away from home? What challenging eating situation can you prepare for? Invite God into the process! He longs to hear from you and will lovingly guide your steps.[58] How might this help you?

_____

_____

_____

> **Extend grace to yourself as you learn this. It takes practice, like riding a bike.**

Try an experiment. Plan three incidences during the next few days to land on a 0 at a time when you normally *aren't* at a 0. To make it fun, you can invite a friend or family member to join you for a meal at that time. It can be a meal out or a meal at home or at a friend's. If you already have a social calendar filled with potential eating occasions, you might want to use those (like buffet after church, holiday dinner, baby shower, etc.). Fill in the chart below to plan your hunger:

What time do you want to get hungry? (Include Day & Time)	Where will you be?	How will you plan for hunger?	Follow Up – How did it go?

---

[58] Psalm 37:23

Respond

What has the Lord shown you today? How would He like you to respond?

_____
_____
_____
_____
_____
_____
_____
_____
_____
_____
_____
_____
_____
_____
_____

LESSON 19

Scripture

Wait for the Lord;
Be strong and take heart, wait for the Lord.

Psalm 27:14 (NIV)

Oh, taste and see that the LORD is good!
Blessed is the man who takes refuge in him!

Psalm 34:8 (NIV)

If the Lord delights in a man's way,
He makes his steps firm,
Though he stumble, he will not fall,
For the Lord upholds him with his hand.

Psalm 37:23-24 (NIV)

Perfectionism

What do you think of when you hear the word "perfect"? You might think of a musical piece performed without one note or rhythm amiss. "Perfect" to you might mean the hum of a masterfully tuned car engine, an artistic flower arrangement, or a melt-in-your-mouth meal. Even the most easy-going person enjoys something of value more fully when it is crafted or performed as close to perfection as possible.

We have learned there is no condemnation in Christ and God's grace is big enough to cover all of our sins. We have studied God's amazing Big T Truth. He is indeed enough for us, ready in every moment of our walk with Him to give us all we need for life and godliness in this world. We readily admit that "nobody is perfect," and yet there is a little t truth that often becomes a stumbling block for us where food and eating and our bodies are concerned.[59]

> **There is no condemnation in Christ and God's grace is big enough to cover *all* of our sins.**

---

[59] Romans 8:1, 2 Peter 1:3

Read the statements below. Which of these resonate with you?

> I will be happy when I have the perfect body.
>
> I will feel content when I am at the perfect weight.
>
> I will lose weight when I do this diet perfectly.
>
> I will lose weight if I do this exercise plan perfectly.

What the magazines and diet books and commercials scream at us is just not true. God knows we won't be perfect! He has created us in His image, He asks us to renew our minds with His truth and longs for us to abide in Him. What a relief to know that we do not have to strive to be perfect in our own strength. It has been said that being perfect before God is like trying to shoot a basketball from earth to a hoop on the moon. It's just not possible! True contentment and peace do not come from striving for perfection.[60]

> **What a relief to know that we do not have to strive to be perfect in our own strength.**

As we have seen, it is important that we confront these little t truths and challenge them with the Big T Truths of God's Word or impressed upon you by listening to the Lord in prayer. A wonderful strategy to do this is to personalize Scripture by inserting your name into the Bible verses you study and then pray through that very verse. This way you are actually using God's own words to pray. The results are powerful! For example:

> *"Humble yourselves therefore under the mighty hand of God,*
>
> *that he may exalt you in due time,*
>
> *casting all your cares upon him,*
>
> *for he cares for you"*
>
> *(1Peter 5:6-7)*

You might pray through this verse like so:

> "Lord Jesus, I want to humble myself before You, before Your mighty hand. I know You will exalt me at the right time. Teach me how to cast my cares upon You. I am so thankful for how much You love me!"

Here is another example:

---

[60] Genesis 1:27, Romans 12:2, John 15:4, Psalm 19:7

© 2019 Heidi Bylsma, www.renewedlifementoring.com. All rights reserved. Printed in the United States of America. No part of this book may be used or reproduced in any matter whatsoever without written permission.

"I have set the Lord always before me.

Because he is at my right hand, I will not be shaken.

Therefore my heart is glad and my tongue rejoices, my body also will rest secure"

(Psalm 16:8-9).

You might pray through this passage like this:

> _Heidi_ will set the Lord always before her. Because You are at her right hand, oh Jesus, she will not be shaken. _Heidi's_ heart will therefore be glad and her tongue will rejoice, her body will also rest secure.

Let's give it a try. Look up the verses below and personalize them for yourself. Listen carefully for God's Big T truths as you do.

2 Corinthians 12:9

_____

_____

2 Corinthians 1:3-4

_____

_____

Lamentations 3:24-26

_____

_____

Isaiah 43:18-19

_____

_____

God's message throughout his Word is clear. He is our strength. He is our Guide, our Rock, the One Who can meet all of our needs. God's strength is made perfect in our weakness! We are to go to Him for everything we need, not strive for perfection that can never be reached in our own power. [61]

You might ask, isn't it true that in order to release all of my extra weight and maintain a healthy size I have to eat perfectly within my God-given 0 to 5 boundaries? Thankfully, the answer is no!

---

[61] 2 Corinthians 12:9

© 2019 Heidi Bylsma, www.renewedlifementoring.com All rights reserved. Printed in the United States of America. No part of this book may be used or reproduced in any matter whatsoever without written permission.

> **He is our strength. He is our Guide, our Rock, the One Who can meet all of our needs. God's strength is made perfect in our weakness!**

Countless of our participants have found that by renewing their minds daily and drawing their strength from God they are able to eat within their boundaries "much of the time" and still release all of their extra weight. Most importantly, they are able to gain the freedom and peace that comes with a renewed mind in Christ about their body and eating. These imperfect participants have discovered that the only thing they can do perfectly in Thin Within or *Fresh Wind, Fresh Desire* is to refuse to give up![62] This *is* the victory! This *is* doing the journey *well!* We like to say, "Doing Thin Within perfectly is being able to be **imperfect** perfectly, by getting up again when I fall and choosing to learn something from my stumble!"

God offers His strength in our weakness. He wants to use our mistakes to teach us more about His truth. Falling "off of the horse" is part of life for us. You can expect to fall, and sometimes to fall often – sometimes really hard—especially at the beginning of your journey with God. But be encouraged! He will not waste anything but will use each fall as a training opportunity for you to grow toward lasting transformation.[63] Review Appendix D for examples.

> **Doing Thin Within *perfectly* is being able to be *imperfect perfectly*, by getting up again when I fall and choosing to learn something from my stumble!**

What has God impressed upon your heart about perfectionism?

_____
_____
_____
_____

How has perfectionism been a stumbling block to you in the past?

_____
_____
_____
_____

---

[62] Phillipians 4:7
[63] Colossians 2:2

© 2019 Heidi Bylsma, www.renewedlifementoring.com. All rights reserved. Printed in the United States of America. No part of this book may be used or reproduced in any matter whatsoever without written permission.

Take a few minutes now to add to your truths. Use the Big T Truths that have been highlighted during today's study.

To Release Weight

There are several strategies that can be used to bring you encouragement as you let go of perfectionism and embrace the training process. Here are some of our favorites:

> **When you struggle or misstep, ask, "What can I thank God for in this situation?" "What is God teaching me through this stumble?"**

1. Text, e-mail, or call a friend. Share a word as simple as "Victory!" when you get back to your 0-5 eating boundaries after a misstep, or share the whole story.

2. Speak truth out loud. Tell yourself that you are God's beloved child and He is training you through this very situation. Say out loud that you are ready to surrender your eating to God once again.

3. Drop a marble in a jar. Prepare a large jar and get a large bunch of marbles at a craft or toy store. Each time you hit the "reset" button on your God-given boundaries or take your thoughts captive, add a marble to the jar. When the jar is full, treat yourself to something you really enjoy with your loving Savior, like a bubble bath, a new scarf, or a walk in the park on a "perfect" day!

4. Practice gratitude. When you struggle or misstep, ask, "What can I thank God for in this situation?" "What is God teaching me through this stumble?" Make a list and thank God for each way that He is transforming you from within.[64] See Appendix D for examples.

5. Create a victory list. Rather than dwell on your mistakes, revel in your victories and remember to thank God for each one. Examples you might include: I ate slowly at dinner three nights this week, I waited until I was hungry to eat the snack I had in my purse, I renewed my mind when tempted, I selected a Whole Body Pleaser instead of a Taste Bud Teaser, I logged on to the FaceBook group and got encouragement, or I stopped eating when satisfied at a restaurant for the first time. You could even include "I stopped the binge before I had eaten the entire bag of cookies!"

6. Make a sticky note wall. Choose the inside of a kitchen cabinet door or another place in your home to celebrate your victories with sticky notes. Each time you hop back "on the horse" with your God-given boundaries jot a few words on a sticky note about the experience.

7. Come up with your own ideas. Be creative as you let go of perfectionism and allow God to transform you from within. Each time you are "imperfect perfectly," choose to learn from the setback and get back up on the horse!

How did it go yesterday with taking food with you in case you got hungry before you could sit down to a carefully thought out meal?

---

[64] Psalm 100:4

How did planning for o go for you? Fill in the fourth column in Lesson 18, on page **100**. What challenges have you faced? What corrections can you make?

Respond

What has the Lord shown you today? How would He like you to respond?

LESSON 20

Scripture

You have made known to me the path of life;
You will fill me with joy in your presence,
With eternal pleasures at your right hand.

Psalm 16:11 (NIV)

How can a young person stay on the path of purity?
By living according to your word.
I seek you with all my heart;
do not let me stray from your commands.

Psalm 119:9-10 (NIV)

I have hidden your word in my heart that I might not sin against You.

Psalm 119:11 (NIV)

It's a Long Trail Ride

Have you ever gone horseback riding, meandered along a beautiful forest path, relished scenery, and experienced the refreshment of being carried along? Horses have minds of their own and, at times, don't much care for the will of their passengers, balking at a water crossing or getting anxious if separated from a favored pasture mate. Beautiful prey animals, horses can be startled into flight mode by a glittery bit of garbage blowing harmlessly in the wind. If the horse "spooks," an inexperienced rider may lose his balance and land on the ground!

> **It is God's great and glorious nature to give. He supplies all we need, day in and day out.**

There are strategies to prevent falling off the horse (other than duct tape ☺). Each time a rider loses his balance, it can be turned into a learning opportunity to evaluate "How did that happen?" and "What can I do differently next time?"

Sometimes on our Thin Within and *Fresh Wind, Fresh Desire* journeys, we are a bit like a horseback rider. A trouble or trial arises, and we find ourselves suddenly unsteady, slipping off, "failing" in our efforts with 0 to 5 eating. This may come as quite a shock, especially when we were doing so well! Has this happened to you? Please describe it on the next page:

_____

_____

_____

_____

Blast from the Past

Going through a rapid-fire series of trials, I experienced a number of challenges with staying on the horse! Specifically, I found myself *craving* peanut butter cookies for the first time in my life! The insecurity caused in my heart and mind by fixating on the storms of my life instead of Jesus, intensified my discontent and agitation. This only enlarged my yearning for cookies. For the life of me, I couldn't figure out why the craving was so strong. I am not proud to say that I gave in quite a lot to that longing. I was often at 0 when I did so. Nevertheless, I began to realize that something was going on deeper than what I could see. My struggle was very much attached to the emotional upheaval in my life. Reaching for home-made peanut butter cookies was my weak attempt to calm and comfort myself.

What was causing this repeated slip off the horse? How could I remedy this? Was my heart rebellious and unwilling to yield to the Lord? I didn't think so, as often I **was** hungry, but why peanut butter cookies when there are lots of wonderful foods I could enjoy?

The Lord knows what is going on in my heart, even when I don't have a clue, so I sat down with my journal, bible, and pen, invited God to shine His light on the situation and asked Him: Why am I craving peanut butter cookies? Is there an ingredient my body needs? Is my mind playing a role? Is my heart?

As silly as it sounds now, I journaled about my earliest memories of freshly baked peanut butter cookies. I can't remember a single day when my mother baked cookies, so it wasn't some sort of longing for my mom (who passed away in 2012).

As I called up the memory, the visual image in my mind included crisscross indentations on each peanut butter cookie, impressed upon the pre-cooked dough with a fork. Fresh out of the oven, I could even see the sugar sprinkled on each delectable, fragrant morsel in my mind.

> **One bite past "satisfied" is not necessarily a *sin* unless you sense conviction from the Holy Spirit. We assert that it isn't the food so much as resisting God's leadership that is the sin issue.**

Where did this memory come from? Prayerfully, I enjoyed remembering and, even as I did (and as I write about it right now), a calm came over me! I stayed with the imagery a bit longer and I was teleported in my mind to the kitchen where I was raised. I was confused, as I had never had any happy memories associated with that kitchen, as it was the location of a lot of abuse and unhappiness.

I let the memory play in my mind and suddenly and quite unexpectedly, there was "Grandma Breit" pulling the next batch of cookies out of the oven. Oh! I hadn't thought of Grandma Breit in years! She was typically a stern task-master and my good memories of her are few and far between, but the rare times she stayed with me while my parents were out of town, if I came home from school and she was pulling cookies out of the oven, I knew all would be well. Grandma would be in a good mood, she would give me cookies, and for a brief hour or two, I knew life would be without turmoil.

God used that memory to show me that **it wasn't the peanut butter cookies** themselves that had a hold on me triggering the craving. It was the emotion that I attached to my earliest memory of freshly baked peanut butter cookies! I was yearning for the calm, the quiet, the affirmation, the relief associated for me with peanut butter cookies. If I saw cookies when Grandma Breit was there, I knew I wasn't in trouble! I knew she wouldn't be cranky! Now, as an adult going through trials, I longed to feel that same peace, calm and relief.

> **It wasn't the cookie so much as the *memory* of peace, calm and "okayness" that I associated with the cookie that called to me.**

I determined to ask the Lord if there are other ways I can bring this sensation into my experience, so I could feel peace, calm, and relief without eating anything. This caused a huge breakthrough for me! I could meet the need I had in a positive, more godly way. It wasn't the cookie so much as the *memory* of peace, calm and "okayness" that I associated with the cookie that called to me.

Observation and correction led me to ask the Lord how I could meet the emotional need in the midst of my trials in other ways. A short list of ideas includes:

- Taking a bath.
- Going on a hike.
- Sitting outside in the sun.
- Getting a massage.

These landed on my list of alternatives to peanut butter cookies to grant myself the restful space I longed for.

Your Turn

Picture a favorite food that would be impossible for you to resist if someone were to put it on a table in front of you, hungry or not. Close your eyes and imagine it. Jot down here, what it is:

_____

Now, call up the earliest (or most relevant) memories you have of the food. Let the memory unfold like a movie in your mind. Describe the scene. What were you feeling when you ate it? Who was present? How did it affect your mood?

_____

_____

_____

_____

_____

_____

What alternatives might supply the emotions that you listed that you have gleaned from eating that particular food in your memory? How could you meet the need in some other way?

_____

_____

_____

_____

OPTIONAL ~ Task 1: Take some time to create a timeline of the favorite food (or beverage) in your life. How old were you, who were you with, what were the circumstances, what associations do you make in your memory between the food/drink and emotions that you *want* to feel? Write these down with your age and the rough guesstimate of the year.

OPTIONAL ~ Task 2: Take time to journal or verbally write gratitudes to the Lord for the people and situations in your life God used to comfort you and encourage you. The goal here is to give credit where credit is due…we may subconsciously reach for a food that we attach to good feelings and happy memories, but we want instead to take time to thank God for the positive emotions, people, situations through which He comforted us. When I do this, the influence of the food or beverage is demystified and less compelling!

It can be tricky to sift through heart, head and physical hunger, but if you, like me, begin to have an inexplicable longing for a food that, while always enjoyable, has never been something at the top of your "yummy" list, ask the Lord to show you if it is the food or the *feeling* you associate with eating that particular food. Ask Him to show you if it still provides that relief today and what you can do differently to meet the need more adequately. When we desire to eat something, it is challenging sometimes to S.T.A.L.L., but if we do, we can ask the Lord questions like these.

© 2019 Heidi Bylsma, www.renewedlifementoring.com. All rights reserved. Printed in the United States of America. No part of this book may be used or reproduced in any matter whatsoever without written permission.

Scripture Snapshot

Read Genesis 4:7 and James 1: 13-15. What do you learn from these verses?

_____

_____

_____

_____

What principle can be gleaned from James 1:13-15 that applies to the temptation we sometimes face to break our eating boundaries?

_____

_____

_____

_____

Use James 1:14-15 to write a progression that fills in the chart provided. The answers are provided in the footnotes.[65]

_____ ⇒ _____ ⇒ _____

Again, one bite past "just enough" is not necessarily a sin unless you sense conviction from the Holy Spirit and ignore it. We assert that it isn't eating the food so much as resisting God's leadership that is the obedience or sin issue. However, most of us can identify with eating so much at one time that we can consider it excessive, greedy, or gluttonous. In what ways has eating more than your body needs resulted in "death" in your past?

_____

_____

_____

_____

---

[65] Desire, sin, death

Refer to Romans 13:14. What are ways we might "make provision for the flesh" in our eating? What desires or emotions have lured you to eat outside of your boundaries?

> **The Holy Spirit is in us to enable us to make good, God-honoring choices.**

Consider two "Events" when you have given in to temptation to eat outside of your boundaries recently. (Don't worry! We will introduce the "Victory List" in Lesson 21 to give equal time to record the wonderful things you and God have partnered together to do on this journey!) Use the chart below to record your thoughts.

In the first column, "**Event**," briefly describe who, what food, when, where, and how you broke your boundaries.

In the "**Lies**" column, jot down what belief (lie or little t truth) fueled the event.

Then, in your mind, review the minutes (or hours) preceding the breaking of your boundaries. Dismantle what happened. Jot down these "**Decision Points Leading Up to the Event**" in the appropriate column. Record here the moments when you could have turned another direction or chosen *not* to make "provision for the flesh."

Finally, in the fourth column, make brief notes about what you could do in the future should you run into the same sort of situation. Include the "Big T Truth" that God wants you to believe.

Event	Lies or "little t truths"	Decision Points Leading Up to the Event	Wisdom for Next Time
(What happened?)	(What did I believe?)	(When could I have turned?)	(What will I believe to be victorious?)

Let's practice thinking God's thoughts after Him. As we renew our minds, we are redirected by His powerful truth. If you have renewed your mind less often since you began this journey because you have been victorious, we urge you to return to the practice on a regular basis. Some of us have experienced a "relapse" by failing to continue our renewing of the mind habit. Learn from our mistakes! Remain prepared for future challenges that are sure to come![66]

To Release Weight – Planning for Trials

It may be an all-inclusive Caribbean cruise with a continuous flow of beverages and mountains of food...

It could be a series of end-of-the-year holidays one after the other complete with cookie exchanges and church potlucks...

It could be a chronic diagnosis with little hope on the horizon for a "normal" life ever again or you might discover your husband's airline frequent flyer account has a companion pass...and it isn't in your name!

Maybe it's a challenging situation at work, difficult family members coming to visit, a house full of sick kids, an expensive car repair or all of the above!

> **Let's practice thinking God's thoughts after Him. As we renew our minds, we are redirected by His powerful truth.**

Whatever it is for you, we *all* can anticipate that challenges *will* come! Maybe you have already experienced victory in surrendering your eating to the Lord and have seen physical, emotional, and spiritual results. Or maybe you are just getting started. But we *all* can press on to draw closer to the Lord by learning to fill our minds with His truth when we are tempted in some way. God's Big T Truth will drain the power out of our little t truths or the lies we have believed.[67]

---

[66] Romans 12:2, Psalm 119:11
[67] John 8:32, Phillipians 3:13

© 2019 Heidi Bylsma, www.renewedlifementoring.com All rights reserved. Printed in the United States of America. No part of this book may be used or reproduced in any matter whatsoever without written permission.

> **God's Big T Truth will drain the power out of our little t truths or the lies we have believed.**

As with a trail ride, our *progress* is the goal. We are not striving for perfection! We are in this for the long haul. When we slip off of the horse in our conscious eating journeys and eat outside of our boundaries—be it with a full-blown binge or a few too many bites past 5—let's not wallow around in the dirt, beating ourselves up. God does not waste anything, and lovingly uses each stumble as a teaching opportunity! Let us dust ourselves off and look at what we can do differently the next time. Read the instructions on the following page before completing the chart.

Think back to the "Look and Learn" ideas discussed in Lessons 9 and 10. Consider what you have observed in the first chart. What two tempting or challenging situations might you face this week? Complete the chart below. Plan now for victory!

Possible Situation	What Could Happen	What I Want to Happen	Evaluate
(Who, what, when, where, why?)	(What lies might I believe?)	(What truth can I believe instead?)	(How did it go? ~ Complete afterwards.)

Respond

What has the Lord shown you today? How would He like you to respond?

LESSON 21

Scripture

*And let the peace of Christ rule in your hearts,
to which indeed you were called in one body.
And be thankful.
Let the word of Christ dwell in you richly,
teaching and admonishing one another in all wisdom,
singing psalms and hymns and spiritual songs,
with thankfulness in your hearts to God.
And whatever you do, in word or deed,
do everything in the name of the Lord Jesus,
giving thanks to God the Father through him.*

Colossians 3:15-17 (ESV)

Mastered by God Alone

In the first phase of *Fresh Wind, Fresh Desire*, as with Thin Within, we enjoy the Freedom Phase—freedom from dieting rules and "good food" and "bad food" lists. We discover we can eat or drink *anything* in moderation and release extra weight.

As we press on, toward Phase 2, what Thin Within calls, the Discernment Phase, we continue in freedom. We learn how to prayerfully practice discernment but with a spirit of adventure! . Lesson 11 introduced what Thin Within calls the Whole Body Pleaser list and the Total Rejects list. We encourage you to continue to add to your lists. You began your Taste Bud Teasers List in Lesson 14. 1 Corinthians 6:12 reads, "All things are lawful for me, but not all things are profitable." We apply this truth by exercising discernment in our eating and drinking, choosing those foods that energize us and make us feel good!

> **Only the Lord Jesus Christ, himself, is to master us.**

Now, looking at the rest of 1 Corinthians 6:12 that says, "All things are lawful for me, but I will not be ***mastered*** by anything," we begin to consider that only the Lord Jesus Christ, himself, is to master us. Not cookies, or pizza, or our favorite salad! This is God's will for us. He desires us to experience peace, freedom, and to be Spirit-led in all things—including our eating. This is the Phase 3, what Thin Within calls the Mastery Phase.

Can you say no to *any* foods—even your favorites? If a certain food is offered to you or available in the house, does 0 to 5 with that food seem an impossible expectation?

To demonstrate that nothing but Jesus has mastery over you, it can be helpful to ask the Lord to show you if he would have you fast a particular food or beverage for a short season—a week or two. If the thought of not having that favorite food or beverage in your life for a few days causes panic, consider it an indication that there may be an inappropriate attachment to that food or beverage. We don't usually find that it is helpful to "outlaw" *whole* groups of foods (like all white flour products) or a specific food for an *indefinite* period of time, unless your doctor feels that you have a health condition that requires abstinence. But it can be helpful to set aside a certain favorite food or beverage for a time. Please ask the Lord to show you His will for you.

What foods are you likely to eat no matter what your hunger number? Are there foods you are likely to select for *every* 0 to 5 eating occasion even though your body might function better with more variety? One 0 to 5 meal after another of brownies until the pan is empty is "permissible," but not beneficial! Do brownies own me? Think about scenarios that challenge you:

- A dish of _____ is on the counter at work and it is impossible to walk by and resist, hungry or not.

- At a Super Bowl party, abstaining from the _____ is beyond you.

At a buffet, these are the foods you want larger portions or seconds of:

_____

_____

What other foods have mastery over you? How do you know?

_____

_____

_____

_____

We want to emphasize that the culprit behind our breaking our eating boundaries **isn't the food**. It is an issue of our **hearts**. In fact, that is one reason why Thin Within and *Fresh Wind, Fresh Desire* might be so challenging for us compared to diets. Sadly, we come face to face with the fact that our hearts seem to bow before favorite foods of all kinds, even when our bodies are suffering from aches in our joints from carrying extra weight. In Lesson 20 we addressed the reasons some foods may seem to have a 'magical hold' on us. Be sure to consider the attachments any foods have to people, feelings, and memories like we discussed.

Thankfully, our God offers us His power through the Holy Spirit living in our bodies—no matter the condition we are in! This is blessedly good news! There is no condemnation for those of us in Christ. There *is*, however, new hope for the future. God is doing a new thing!

Right now, still your heart and mind. Use the following prayer (or one of your own) to invite God to show you what He might want you to do in response to what He has shown you.

© 2019 Heidi Bylsma, www.renewedlifementoring.com. All rights reserved. Printed in the United States of America. No part of this book may be used or reproduced in any matter whatsoever without written permission.

> *Dear Lord, I know that You call me not to be mastered by anything except You alone. If I am honest, I know that there are some foods and beverages that master me whether I am at a 0 or not. Even the thought of giving them up bothers me a bit, to be honest. Lord, please show me what to do especially in light of the admonishment in 1 Corinthians 6:12 that I am not to be mastered by anything. I sense that my fists are tightly gripped around these foods and beverages and I long to feel the peace that comes from letting go. Please show me how, in Jesus' Name, Amen.*

Be silent for a few moments right now. He wants to respond to your request. We wait for Him to lovingly impress His answer on our hearts and that we might gain clarity about what we should do. Write your thoughts here:

_____

_____

_____

_____

If God directs you to let go of a food or beverage for a week or two, after you have obeyed Him about it, evaluate what He would have you do next. He may urge you to continue fasting for another week or two. Or He may lead you to renew your mind about the food or drink as you integrate it back into your life in moderation. This time, you will be exercising submission to His leadership so that nothing masters you except for Christ! When doing so, ask yourself if that food still has the hold on you it once did. It is always possible to set it aside again should the issue resurface.

To Release Weight

It is rewarding to see our thinking change, isn't it? One participant shared with joy that when she and her young son had some unexpected time to spend together, instead of turning on the TV, which she confessed has often resulted in mindlessly eating outside of her boundaries, she and her son enjoyed playing a board game together. She has begun to think differently! She enjoyed precious time with her son instead of maintaining the destructive habit of mindless eating. By taking the time to renew her mind with her truth cards, God List, and PraiseFest, her *desires* had changed! What victory! Over time she is being transformed by the renewing of her mind, just as Romans 12:2 promises. The fresh wind of the Holy Spirit at work in her life has brought fresh desire.

> **By taking the time to renew her mind with her truth cards, God List, and PraiseFest, her *desires* had changed! What victory!**

A wonderful strategy for this participant and any of us is to write down our victories as we continue on this path. We call this a "Victory List" or "Victory Journal." Whenever you make a choice that you *know* is out of character for you and indicative that God is at work doing a new thing, jot it down. Every baby step is worthy to be included on your Victory List or in your Victory Journal.

- Did you stop eating before you would have in the past?
- Did you want food, but remind yourself that you weren't hungry yet and busy yourself with another activity?
- Were you emotional and, instead of plowing through a sleeve of Girl Scout cookies, chose to call a friend to encourage *her* heart?
- Have you previously focused obsessively on the bathroom scale multiple times each day and haven't hopped on it for a week?

We encourage you to include *any* positive emotional, spiritual, *or* physical changes you have experienced on your Victory List. If you are spending time in God's Word, are growing in intimacy with the Savior, are processing emotions with God's help instead of numbing them with food—all of these are worthy to include. And if you see physical changes in your body you can definitely add those too. For example, "My mind feels at peace this week," or "I slipped into a smaller pair of jeans today!"

Think back to when you began this study. What are some of the victories you have experienced—big or small? See if you can come up with at least ten and list them here.

Victory List

1. _____

2. _____

3. _____

4. _____

© 2019 Heidi Bylsma, www.renewedlifementoring.com. All rights reserved. Printed in the United States of America. No part of this book may be used or reproduced in any matter whatsoever without written permission.

5. _____

_____

_____

6. _____

_____

_____

7. _____

_____

_____

8. _____

_____

_____

9. _____

_____

_____

10. _____

_____

_____

One of the joys that can come of creating a list or journal dedicated specifically to recording your victories is that you can use it to pray, giving thanks and gratitude to God. This is another great way to renew your mind with the fact that He is doing a new thing and completing the good work that He has begun in you! When you are feeling discouraged and think you are not getting anywhere, pull out your victory list/journal and read all that God has done and thank him again! (Thank Him that you are free from dieting forever, too!) Getting our eyes off of our own performance and back on to our wonderful King and Lord, is a perfect antidote to emotions that often lead us to the kitchen.

Let's try it now. Read through your Victory List above and say each one out loud to God in prayer form. For example, "Thank you God, for the wonderful time I had playing a game with my son instead of turning to my usual habit of TV and snacks! I see that you are changing me!" *When you have done that, check this box.* ☐

Now that you have spent time thanking God for the way He is at work in you, what value do you think a Victory List/Journal may have for you? Will you give it a try for a week and see?

_____
_____
_____
_____

Respond

What has the Lord shown you today? How would He like you to respond?

_____
_____
_____
_____
_____
_____
_____
_____
_____
_____
_____

LESSON 22

Scripture

Such a person feeds on ashes;
a deluded heart misleads him;
he cannot save himself, or say,
"Is not this thing in my right hand a lie?"

Isaiah 44:20 (NIV)

The Power of Forgiveness ~ Heidi's Story

When my kids were young, I faced daily challenges with one of my kids about homeschooling. It seemed like we were constantly at odds. My own mother had been unstable. The hurdles with my child triggered painful issues from my past. My child had no idea that many of my reactions were based on my personal history that had nothing to do with the present. For a long time, neither did I.

For instance, when we had a confrontation, I felt trapped just like I did when my mom yelled and threw things so many years before. It was as if I was ten years old again. I felt as though I was walking on eggshells—just like with my mom, trying so hard *not* to set my child off.

> **A fog seemed to lift. I found myself sitting in the bathroom with a spoon in one hand and a container of chocolate frosting in the other....**

I remember feeling like I couldn't do anything right. I felt like God must have made a colossal mistake when He gave *me* to my child to be the Mom!

I often ran to food in secret on those difficult days. Yes . . . I *snuck* food! Looking back now, I see how odd my behavior was. One day, after a particularly challenging interaction, a fog seemed to lift. As the curtain parted, I found myself sitting in the bathroom with a spoon in one hand and a container of chocolate frosting in the other. My eyes were opened.

*What am I doing in here? Why am I sneaking? **I** am the grown up! What in the world do I think this frosting will do for me?*

> **It was as if eating in hiding was going to somehow "get back at" my mother.**

It is obvious now that my thinking was off kilter. In those moments of hiding I was holding on to the same thoughts that I had when I was a child. In my pain and confusion, I thought . . . *"I'll show them! I will eat what I want when they don't know about it!"* It was as if eating in hiding was going to somehow "get back at" my mother. I realized that I was doing the same thing with my child! A boatload of lies and little t truths were accompanying me into that bathroom. I am so grateful that God opened my eyes to how crazy my behavior was.

Have you ever had a moment of clarity like this? Does my story resonate with you right now? Do you sense deep in your heart that you *need* to have a moment like this? Write your thoughts here. Use another sheet of paper if you need more space.

___

___

___

___

___

___

___

___

Many Thin Within participants can identify in some way with behavior like mine on my roughest homeschooling days. For some, it is a reaction to a spouse trying to control their eating and weight. For others, it might be a reaction to an unruly child, a physical challenge or illness, or a difficult person at church, school, or work. It may be a reaction, like mine, that had to do with painful past events. What these situations often have in common, is the way we react by grasping for lies or little t truths instead of being rooted firmly in God's Big T Truth.

As a child, before I knew the Lord, I developed a tendency to turn to food to be my comfort. This may not be the case for everyone, but often we establish our habit of going to food when we aren't hungry in response to stressful situations of some kind—as a child, teenager, college student or career person. In fact, many of us have developed a pattern of turning to food when *any* emotion hits us: happiness, sadness, anxiety, excitement, boredom, insecurity, loneliness, confusion, etc.

> **Exalting God is a powerful antidote to pride, which is at the root of most sin!**

What is Your Story?

Many Thin Within participants and readers of *Fresh Wind Fresh Desire*, had wonderful childhoods. But if you are one of those who had difficulty in your childhood, please take a moment to write about it here. Prayerfully ask God to give you *His* thoughts about it. He longs to hear from you and to guide you through this! See if you can notice the value food had for you during that time. Use additional paper as needed.

Now think back to challenges you might have had in other seasons of your life, including the one you are currently in. What life events might fall into the category of "difficult memories?" Again, note the place food had/has for you in these situations:

Can you think of any ways in which these circumstances of the past (even if only 6 months or a year ago) might be impacting you today? How?

_____

Re-read what you have written. Do you see any little t truths or lies that you have believed that are in connection with what you recorded? What are they?

_____

What Big T Truths might God want to speak over you about those challenges and subsequent little t truths or lies that you have rehearsed? Remember that a Big T Truth doesn't have to be a quoted bible verse but can be something you sense that God would want you to believe based on his character and his love and gentleness with you. It will never contradict Scripture.

_____

_____

_____

_____

_____

_____

_____

_____

To Release Weight ~ More from Heidi

I had an accountability partner once who knew me well. Any time I gave in to temptation and broke my 0 to 5 eating boundaries, she knew to ask me "Who do you need to forgive?" It caused me to wonder . . . why would I want to blast through boundaries that had fallen for me in pleasant places[68]? In my case, it seemed to happen when I was stirred up inside about a wrong done to me, whether it was perceived or real. Old habits that I learned in my youth resurfaced when I felt wounded or misunderstood.

> **Forgiveness is a decision to *act*—not an emotion.**

As I began to keep short accounts and do the work of forgiving more readily, I found that my overreacting to emotional "triggers" in present time diminished and I was much more willing and able to stay within my eating boundaries. Does that sound amazing? I was surprised, too.

Continuing Your Story

*Bear with each other
and forgive one another if any of you has a grievance against someone.
Forgive as the Lord forgave you.*

Colossians 3:13

---

[68] Psalm 16:6

How has the Lord forgiven you?

_____

_____

_____

_____

> **Although we are called to forgive, it is not easy by any means! Be gentle with yourself and prayerfully ask God to give you the grace to forgive as Jesus has forgiven you.**

Is there anyone *you* need to forgive who has come to mind? We often are called to forgive again and again as it is for me with my mom who left to be with Jesus in 2012, and my child who is now an adult. If you are like me in this, will you do that now, "telling on them" to God? Be specific about what they did to you, how old you were, how you felt, and how it impacted you.

Remember that forgiveness is a decision to act—not an emotion. Also realize that although we are called to forgive, it is not easy by any means! Be gentle with yourself and prayerfully ask God to give you the grace to forgive as Jesus has forgiven you. He longs to free us of these grievances and offers us His strength, and His peace that passes all understanding. Below, write out "forgiveness phrases" for anyone you need to forgive.

For example, "I forgive my Dad for being so critical of me when I was a child" or "I forgive my best friend for pulling away from me when I needed her the most." Use additional paper and be as comprehensive as possible.

_____

_____

_____

_____

_____

_____

_____

_____

Final Thoughts from Heidi

Forgiveness, Gratitude and Praise are the three cornerstones of breakthrough in my personal Thin Within journey. This is because it is impossible to continue to exalt myself and grasp for more food when I humble myself and renew my mind through forgiveness, gratitude, and praise. Exalting God is a powerful antidote to pride, which is at the root of most sin!

Bring it Home

Today has been a challenging lesson to read and complete. (It's also been difficult for me to write. ☺) Maybe you want to set your workbook down and not complete this lesson. I understand. But if you come back to it and prayerfully work through it, I promise that shackles will be broken. Freedom rings! Do you remember the God List and PraiseFest? Take 10 minutes to add to your God List and/or to Praise the King of Kings. End today's session with praise! *Check this box when you have done that.* ☐

Respond

What has the Lord shown you today? How would He like you to respond?

_____

_____

_____

_____

_____

_____

_____

_____

_____

_____

© 2019 Heidi Bylsma, www.renewedlifementoring.com All rights reserved. Printed in the United States of America. No part of this book may be used or reproduced in any matter whatsoever without written permission.

LESSON 23

Scripture

*You will keep in perfect peace
those whose minds are steadfast,
because they trust in You.*

Isaiah 26:3 (NIV)

*And the peace of God, which transcends all understanding,
will guard your hearts and minds in Christ Jesus.*

Philippians 4:7 (NLT)

Maintenance

What a journey this is! Our study of *Fresh Wind, Fresh Desire*, may be ending soon, but we head into the future with a new mindset, a new outlook, a new set of transforming truths and tools that God will use to continue to change us!

Are you closer to Him than when you began? Have you taken a hard look at why you do the things you do? Seen a shift in your thinking? Or perhaps you are just beginning to get a glimpse of God's plan for you. Whether you have released weight or not, *all* of us have been touched and changed in some way over these past weeks by God's amazing Big T truths. Once you dive into His Word it's impossible not to be! His powerful Word expresses His constant, unchangeable, and boundless love for us.[69]

Let's take a look at what the world often says life might be like when you have reached your "goal weight." What do you think?

In order to maintain my new, smaller size I will:

- Eat within my boundaries almost *perfectly* every day.

- Come up with and stick to a *rigorous* exercise plan.

- Be fine with giving up certain foods and drinks.

- Keep up a body that looks like a fashion model.

- Relish only "healthy" and "good" foods. *Never* have any "junk" food.

---

[69] Isaiah 43:19, Matthew 11:28, Hebrews 4:12, Philippians 4:7

© 2019 Heidi Bylsma, www.renewedlifementoring.com. All rights reserved. Printed in the United States of America. No part of this book may be used or reproduced in any matter whatsoever without written permission.

Wait a minute . . . Is this what God wants for us?

Remember in Lesson 2, we saw a list of earthly and eternal values that we can pursue. Keeping our bodies "looking good," is a worldly quest. While there is nothing wrong with taking care of ourselves so that the temple of God—our bodies, which He has graciously entrusted to us—are as healthy and function as well as possible, we can put far too *much* value on being thin or fit, failing to see that we are bowing to the "idol of skinny" or the "idol of good health." As with our eating, we want to maintain a godly balance. These "earth suits" are temporary![70]

> **Jesus made us to yearn for intimacy with *Him* and the abundant life He has promised us.**

Jesus made us to yearn for intimacy with *Him* and the abundant life He has promised us. We desire peace with who we are, peace with our weaknesses, with the difficult situations in our lives, with our bodies, with our Sovereign God. Freedom from compulsive eating, dieting or exercising in response to emotions or situations is now within our grasp. Eating for reasons other than physical hunger, we no longer jam the proverbial "square peg in a round hole." Recognizing that only God can fill the God-shaped void in our hearts will help us reject turning to food, which satisfies only *physical* hunger—not *heart* hunger. That's the bottom line. That's the finish line. *Living* there *is* the "other side." That *is* the maintenance plan![71]

> **Freedom from compulsive eating, dieting or exercising in response to emotions or situations is now within our grasp.**

Take a minute to think about your heart's deepest cry—beyond the size of your jeans or the menu at your favorite restaurant. Ask God to show you what you yearn for Him to provide. Use this time to cry out to Him and write down your thoughts here:

_____

_____

_____

_____

_____

_____

---

[70] 1 Timothy 4:8
[71] John 10:10, Psalm 29:11, Isaiah 26:3, Psalm 119:165

© 2019 Heidi Bylsma, www.renewedlifementoring.com All rights reserved. Printed in the United States of America. No part of this book may be used or reproduced in any matter whatsoever without written permission.

A Word from Christina on "Maintenance"

When I first started to apply the principles I learned in Thin Within to my own life I desperately wanted to talk with someone who had already found the peace and freedom with eating and their body that I wanted. I couldn't imagine that after years and years of dieting, over-exercising and ups and downs on the scale that there really was such a thing. The good news is that there is! There really is! We are not talking about perfection by any means. We will all be a work in progress until the day we meet Jesus in person. But there is beautiful, not-of-this-world hope for the peace and freedom we crave, and it's offered to each and every one of us.[72] Here is what "maintenance" looks like to me:

> **Only God can fill the God-shaped void in our hearts.**

1. My relationship with God is deeper and more intimate than ever.

2. I depend on God and submit to His will knowing that change comes from the inside, from His work in my life.

3. My hope is in God who can do all things. My hope is *not* in me!

4. I praise Him and exalt Him, getting my eyes off me and on **Him**.

5. I renew my mind, filling my thoughts with Big T Truths, crowding out the little t truths and lies that I used to believe.

6. When I struggle with a difficult situation or emotion I go to God first knowing that food will never meet the needs I have.

7. When I stumble and eat outside of my boundaries I don't feel hopeless anymore. There is no condemnation in Christ, so I again wait for physical hunger and continue on in my journey.

8. I eat smaller portions more naturally now and I spend much less money on food.

9. The clothes in my closet fit comfortably. No more hours spent wrestling with what to wear anymore or obsessing over the scale.

10. I used to spend so much time worrying about what I would eat, what I would wear and how I looked. Now I feel comfortable in my own skin and can spend that time thinking of much more important things!

> **My relationship with God is deeper and more intimate than ever.**

11. I eat a variety of foods in moderate portions that cause my body to feel good physically. I know that my body needs good fuel to function as well as it can.

---

[72] Psalm 25:5, Psalm 65:5, Psalm 119:74, Isaiah 40:31

12. I don't strive to look like a magazine model anymore. I am fearfully and wonderfully made and have accepted my body with all of its imperfections.

13. I recognize the red flags along the way. For example, if my clothes aren't fitting comfortably, or I find myself mastered by a specific food I know that something isn't right with my heart and I take it to God.

14. I view my mistakes and stumbles as learning opportunities and become stronger as God teaches me.

> **I view my mistakes and stumbles as learning opportunities and become stronger as God teaches me.**

15. With less preoccupation with myself, I am able to minister to others and love them well as I am called by God to do.

How About You?

Which of these thoughts from Christina bring you hope? Which encourage you? Circle or underline the ones that do.

What might God be saying to you about *your* maintenance plan? What hopes can you lay before Him? Write your thoughts here as a prayer:

_____
_____
_____
_____
_____

What Big T Truths has God shown you today? Take a moment to write out any new truths in your cards or lists that will bring courage and inspiration to you about your Thin Within journey. *Mark this box when you have done so.* ☐

Sometime today, review any of your truth cards for five minutes. *Check this box when you do so.* ☐

Pick an additional activity to spend five additional minutes doing from the following list. (Circle) the one you choose and mark the box when you have completed it. ☐

1. Add to your God List.

2. Have a PraiseFest.

3. Add to your Victory List.

4. Practice S.T.A.L.L. at least once today.

5. Etc. _____

To Release Weight – "Margin of 5"

The principles of Thin Within are *simple*—but not *easy*. We eat when we are physically hungry and stop when our bodies are satisfied. We hope in Him and fill our minds with His Truth as He transforms us from the inside. Certainly, one of the biggest changes in our thinking is realizing that it doesn't take much food to sustain us!

Are you releasing weight? Consider your definition for "enough" or 5. Those who define 5 as **no longer hungry**, stop eating at the "*near*" end of what we call the "Margin of 5." By contrast, the "*far*" end of the Margin of 5 is the place where we eat **as much as we can** before we have to call it a 6. The difference in the amount of food eaten in this margin may be equivalent to another fist-sized portion of food! If we continue to eat to the far end of the 5 margin, we may struggle to release our weight. If you don't see more space inside your clothes by now, consider the "Margin of 5" as a possible explanation. Are you stopping at the *near* end of the 5 margin or at the *far* end of the 5 margin? Somewhere in between?

_____

_____

_____

_____

Congratulations if you have released weight. A word of caution: Be aware of complacency or pride once you reach your God-given size. The biggest pitfall that Thin Within veterans often share is pride. Perhaps the most important thing about "maintenance" in Thin Within is to maintain what we did as we released the weight: keep studying, praying, tracking *victories*, observing and correcting, creating and using God List and PraiseFest, etc., **Maintain a good mind renewal habit.** When we stop renewing our minds with truth, look for counterfeit "fixes" for the needs of our hearts, puff up with pride when people compliment our weight loss, then our boundaries may begin to slip and the old lies begin to surface.[73]

> **When we stop renewing our minds with truth, look for counterfeit "fixes" for the needs of our hearts, puff up with pride when people compliment our weight loss, then our boundaries may begin to slip and the old lies begin to surface.**

---

[73] 2 Corinthians 12:9, Matthew 19:22

© 2019 Heidi Bylsma, www.renewedlifementoring.com. All rights reserved. Printed in the United States of America. No part of this book may be used or reproduced in any matter whatsoever without written permission.

A Long, Slow, Slide ~ Heidi's Story

> We are needy people. God promises to be strong in our weakness! With our hand firmly planted in His, nothing is impossible.

2006 to 2007 I released 100 pounds using Thin Within principles. For years I maintained my God-given size and then, in May of 2014, after a strenuous hike—one of the last I planned to take in preparation for a bucket-list back-packing trip at Machu Picchu in Peru—I began experiencing incredible pain throughout my torso, chest and back. Unknown to me and to doctors who were confounded by my symptoms, a staph infection was feasting on five of my vertebrae.

The removal of my gallbladder didn't solve the problem, of course. It only made everything worse as I continued to be in horrible pain as before, only now the discomfort from the surgery and adjusting to life without a gallbladder kept me from eating very much. Without proper nourishment for two months, my body struggled to fight off the infection that still remained undetected, even while I grew increasingly emaciated. In early July of 2014, the staph infection caused two vertebrae to collapse and I suddenly lost my ability to walk unassisted. An emergency, seven-hour back surgery, complete with an "installation" of titanium rods and pins in my back and tons of opiate painkillers, followed. I was a mess. The last thing I cared about was 0 to 5 eating or my "natural, God-given healthy size." I wanted to be able to walk again!

> I was "bingeing" in my head. In essence, I was "renewing my mind," but instead of with *Truth*, my mind was being wall-papered with *lies* and destructive thoughts.

Previously, when I experienced a trial, I reverted to old coping behaviors from my pre-2006 days—from before I released weight. I processed my emotions with food, was gently corrected by the Holy Spirit, would renew my mind, and get back in the saddle again with 0 to 5 eating without much damage. Now, as intravenous antibiotics and stronger opiate painkillers began to do their jobs, I began to think of eating again. At the hospital for three weeks, they insisted!

Now, during the most frightening trial of my life, I began to have all the thoughts that usually accompanied overeating in response to challenges, but I wasn't *able* to act on my thoughts by overeating. It still hurt to eat, but not to think about food! In fact, I thought a **lot** about what I would love to eat, how much, how wonderful it would be, how good it would make me feel, and how much I "deserved" it for all I was putting up with. One could say I was "bingeing" in my head. It was like I was "renewing my mind," but instead of with Truth, my mind was being wall-papered with *lies* and destructive thoughts. I didn't recognize the harm as I did previously because I couldn't **act** on my thoughts. There were no physical consequences to thinking about food to draw my attention to the condition of my heart and mind. Mind renewal had stopped abruptly in May when I got so sick. In six months, you can sow a lot of seeds of destructive thinking.

Over the next year, I began to eat more like my "normal" 0 to 5 self. I was told I needed to *gain* weight! (That's a first!) I didn't realize that I slowly started to slide, acting subtly on the thoughts that I had rehearsed in my mind for the first six months of my recovery. Like the proverbial frog in the pot of water on the stove who boils to death, I didn't notice that I was slowly heading in to "danger." I could talk about mind renewal with clients and in Thin Within webinars. My mind had *been* renewed, right? No need to carve out time for that now. I had physical therapy and life with new physical challenges to adjust to! I didn't realize how damaged my metabolism was as well.

> **It still hurt to eat, but not to think about food! In fact, I thought a *lot* about what I would love to eat, how much, how wonderful it would be, how good it would make me feel, and how much I "deserved" it for all I was putting up with.**

By the time Christmas of 2015 came and went, I noticed there was less "space" in the jeans I had been wearing for years. Evening dessert "splurges" and drinking sugar-filled beverages outside of 0 and 5 (something I never struggled with before) had become routine. How did this happen? I rarely use a scale. But I decided a reality test might be appropriate. BUSTED. I had been on a long, slow, slide back into doing my own thing, my own way, fueled by lies.

> **Mind renewal had stopped abruptly in May when I got so sick. In six months, you can sow a lot of seeds of destructive thinking.**

I was a casualty of the war of pride, apathy, and rehearsing lies. I am grateful there is no condemnation in Christ. Why God would continue to allow me to keep on reaching out to others in the Thin Within ministry, even while being so hypocritical is demonstrative of His amazing grace. Glad that the Spirit of God has shown me the truth, I am back committed to a process of renewing my mind. I have an accountability partner who is helping me stay on track. I have a prayer partner who is praying constantly for me. I am so grateful for another chance. I see that I must always be on guard against pride.

> **I had been on a long, slow, slide back into doing my own thing, my own way, fueled by lies.**

Respond

What has the Lord shown you today? How would He like you to respond?

_____

_____

© 2019 Heidi Bylsma, www.renewedlifementoring.com. All rights reserved. Printed in the United States of America. No part of this book may be used or reproduced in any matter whatsoever without written permission.

LESSON 24

Scripture

The Lord is my strength and my shield,
my heart trusts in Him, and He helps me.
My heart leaps for joy, and with my song I praise Him.

Psalm 28:7 (NLT)

Let the message of Christ dwell among you richly,
as you teach and admonish one another with all wisdom
through psalms, hymns and songs from the Spirit,
singing to God with gratitude in your hearts.

Colossians 3:16 (NIV)

The Lord lives! Praise be to my rock!
Exalted be my God, the rock, my Savior!

2 Samuel 22:47 (NIV)

Celebration

We are here! It is the last day of this study. Today will be a day of celebration. We will set aside a special time to praise and worship our beautiful Savior for what He has done and continues to do in our lives. Whether or not you have released weight, whether or not you feel that you have really grasped and put into practice the principles of Thin Within there is still reason to rejoice! God is working in you. He is doing something new! He has promised to complete the good work He is doing.[74]

> **We never have to step on a scale again as long as we continue to prayerfully respond to our body's hunger numbers.**

There are dozens of reasons to love the Thin Within approach, not the least of which is we no longer have to worry about what is served when we are out to dinner or visiting with friends. We don't have to avoid any food or beverage, but merely plan for our hunger and be mindful to respond to our body's needs.

---

[74] Isaiah 43:19, Philippians 1:6

© 2019 Heidi Bylsma, www.renewedlifementoring.com. All rights reserved. Printed in the United States of America. No part of this book may be used or reproduced in any matter whatsoever without written permission.

One of the wonderful things about this is if we continue to renew our minds, wait for physical hunger, stop eating when we are physically satisfied, and apply Thin Within's Keys to Conscious Eating, we will maintain our natural God-given size once we have landed there. In fact, we don't even need to be concerned so much with "How much should I weigh?" *The way that we know we are at our natural, God-given size is by consistently applying the Keys to Conscious Eating and eating 0 to 5. When we stop getting smaller and start to maintain, we know we are there.* We never have to step on a scale again as long as we continue to prayerfully respond to our body's physical signals for hunger and enough. The "maintenance program" is the same as what we do to release weight. What a blessing this is! What freedom and peace there is in this glorious future for us!

> **Perfection isn't the point! We don't have to be perfect! We just press on. This is sanctification. It is progressive and we will be taking baby steps forward for the rest of our lives.**

We really can do this for the rest of our lives. This is one reason why we encourage participants again and again to know that perfection isn't the point! We don't have to be perfect! We just press on. This is sanctification. It is progressive, and we will be taking baby steps forward for the rest of our lives. Let's get back on the horse. Push the reset button. We wait for physical hunger and move on that very moment, ready to receive the teaching that God has for us in the midst of our stumbling. Praise God for the amazing way He has made us and for the plans He has set before us. We were not made for fear, anxiety and condemnation! We were made for freedom, peace, for pleasant boundaries and to seek a deeper relationship with the God of the galaxies and all that exists Who created us to worship Him.[75]

Let's praise and worship God together right now. Take out your God list and pray through it to God, lifting up His holy name. Thank Him for who He is in your life, and for who you are because of Him! Renew your mind with the truth that this life is not about us. It's about our marvelous, all-powerful, incredibly amazing God and His purposes and plans. Have you started your Gratitude Journal or Gratitude List? If so, pull it out now and praise God through each thankful statement. If not, begin one today! You may want to put on a favorite praise song or sing one out loud. Close your eyes and breathe Him in . . . allow your praises to float up to heaven and just *be* with Him, even for just a few minutes. Be present with Him. Open your heart to Him. His arms are open wide![76]

> **We were made for freedom, peace, for pleasant boundaries and to seek a deeper relationship with the God of the stars and sky Who created us to worship**

---

[75] Philippians 3:13-15, Jeremiah 29:11, Romans 8:1, Psalm 16:6
[76] 1 Chronicles 16:25, Psalm 9:2, Psalm 28:7, Psalm 59:17, Isaiah 25:1, 2 Corinthians 1:3, Ephesians 1:3

© 2019 Heidi Bylsma, www.renewedlifementoring.com All rights reserved. Printed in the United States of America. No part of this book may be used or reproduced in any matter whatsoever without written permission.

Check this box after you have done a PraiseFest or a Gratitude session (or both!):

Let's spend some quiet time now in reflection. Be sure to ask God into your thoughts so that His Spirit can teach and encourage you. What have you learned about God through this study?

_____
_____
_____
_____
_____
_____
_____

What have you learned about yourself?

_____
_____
_____
_____
_____
_____
_____

What have you learned about your body?

_____
_____
_____
_____
_____
_____
_____

What changes have you seen in your eating? Are you less driven by food?

_____
_____

© 2019 Heidi Bylsma, www.renewedlifementoring.com. All rights reserved. Printed in the United States of America. No part of this book may be used or reproduced in any matter whatsoever without written permission.

If we are more present in the moments of our lives rather than running mindlessly from one thing to the next in our busyness we will be likely to be more present with our eating and food. How is this statement true for you?

To Release Weight

But what about those of us who haven't released *any* weight yet? What if you are just beginning to allow God's Big T truths and the Keys to Conscious Eating sink into your heart and mind? Perhaps you have taken the first steps in this journey and haven't seen a whole lot of visible change yet. Don't worry! Take heart. Just the fact that you are still here, completing the last day of this study shows that God is at work in you.

Here is one more strategy that might be an encouragement to you. We call it "This Moment." Have you had one really good moment today in your journey? Perhaps you waited for physical hunger to have breakfast this morning. Or you ate more slowly than you usually do. Did you eat a food that you enjoy? Maybe your best moment is now—renewing your mind and praising God during this study. Imagine that one really good moment as a beautiful bead on a string.

Next, try to be aware of another moment as you walk through your day. Can you choose your donut from the lounge at work and save it for later? Can you renew your mind with a truth card or two while waiting in line at the pharmacy? Can you thank God for that unexpected hug you received from a friend? Imagine that moment as another sparkling bead and add it to your string. Do you have a picture in your mind of this string of beads? (Maybe you want to actually string together a real necklace or bracelet for one day just to see tangible proof

> **This journey is not about perfection—far from it! It's about a steady moment-by-moment focus on God's truth *throughout* each day.**

of God's work in your day!) Don't worry about the moments you have stumbled in between. God will use those too. Remember that He wastes nothing![77]

As you "string" together one victory after another you will see that this journey is not about perfection as we have said before—far from it! It's about a steady moment-by-moment focus on God's truth throughout each day. Looking and learning, we grow along the way, even from our mistakes. Take note of even "small" victories in your Victory List or Victory Journal. We choose to walk along a path that moves forward regardless of detours and pitfalls. We walk hand in hand with our loving Savior who promises to protect us, provide for us, strengthen us and even carry us along the way. Be encouraged! Know that you are on the right track. God is right beside you! Sling that backpack of Big T Truths and Keys to Conscious Eating on your back and be on your way.

Your journey has just begun! ☺ There is a Fresh Wind and a Fresh Desire. Raise your sails and catch it!

Respond

What has the Lord shown you today? How would He like you to respond?

_____

_____

_____

_____

_____

_____

_____

_____

_____

_____

_____

_____

_____

_____

_____

[77] Psalm 103:1-5

APPENDIX A

What are "Renewing Your Mind Recipes"?

In this section, Christina Motley, Thin Within participant, coach, and expert on renewing her mind, has provided a wonderful smorgasbord of tools you can incorporate into your daily life as a practice of renewing your mind about your body, food, eating, God, your identity – about *anything*, really! This is a crucial aspect of victory in this journey. Treat the options here as a "buffet" where you don't have to worry about "overeating"! ☺ There are a number of options from which you can choose, depending on the amount of time you have available. Enjoy!

SCRIPTURE:

*"Do not conform to the pattern of this world,
but be transformed by the renewing of your mind.
Then you will be able to test and approve what God's
will is – his good, pleasing and perfect will."*

Romans 12:2 (NIV)

INGREDIENTS:[78]

The Bible

Gratitude List	God List	Victory List
Sticky Note Wall	Marble Jar	Truth Cards
Truth Journaling	PraiseFest	Prayer Journaling
Thin Within books	Prayer Partner	Sound Cloud files
Personalizing Scripture	Prayer Walking	I Deserve a Donut
Praying Through Scripture	Original Thin Within videos	Bible-centered devotionals

---

[78] For further description or explanation of any "menu items" for renewing your mind, please visit our OriginalThinWithin YouTube channel, our Sound Cloud channel, or our blog at http://www.thinwithin.org/blog/ Just do a search and you are likely to find that what you are looking for will pop up.

© 2019 Heidi Bylsma, www.renewedlifementoring.com All rights reserved. Printed in the United States of America. No part of this book may be used or reproduced in any matter whatsoever without written permission.

Renewing-the-Mind Recipes

ONE-HOUR PLAN:

1. **Set the stage:** Prepare for a special time with God:

    - **Do you like to be outside?** Take a hike with Jesus or meet Him at a beautiful park. How about your back yard (on a blanket on the lawn), a patio, or a front porch?

    - **Or do you like to be inside?** Choose a favorite spot in your home, perhaps a cozy couch with a warm quilt if it's cold outside. Light a candle and put on background music that you enjoy.

    Whatever location you choose, put away all distractions, and then invite God to be with you. Picture Him right there with you – walking by your side or sitting with you. He has been looking forward to your invitation!

2. **Praise and Worship:** If you like music, choose a praise song that's meaningful to you. Close your eyes and listen, or sing along with it aloud. Let the truth of the words wash over and sink into you as you relax and nestle into His presence. Next, have a PraiseFest! Pray through your God List out loud as you lift up praises to Him about who He is. To complete your PraiseFest, pray through a Psalm or a passage from Isaiah. If you like, spend some time (on your knees, if you're able) in worship to your mighty King. Remember to thank Him for who He is and for drawing you near to Him today!

3. **Thanksgiving:** Take some time to thank God for the many blessings He has given you. Thank Him for everything and anything you can think of, from the warm socks on your feet to the snuggle you received from your child or grandchild yesterday! Pull out your Gratitude List or Gratitude Journal, and use it to thank God for specific things. Be sure to thank Him for your body and that you are fearfully and wonderfully made. Take out your Victory List, your Sticky Note Wall, or your Marble Jar. Use these tools to thank God for all that He is doing in your life and in your heart! Add to them if more ideas come to mind while you're thanking Him!

4. **Big-T Truth:** Choose one or more resources to bring God's truth to your heart today. Here are a few choices: Bible passages, Truth Cards, a flip-calendar of Bible verses, past Truth Journaling, past Journaled Prayers, *Hunger Within* by Judy Halliday, *I Deserve a Donut* or *Taste for Truth* by Barb Raveling, a Bible-centered devotional, or the *Thin Within: Fresh Wind, Fresh Desire* workbook. Ask the Holy Spirit to open your heart to be able to receive His Word, and to speak to you during this time. Fill your mind with Scripture, and journal or speak aloud the Big-T truths that touched your heart today. Talk to God about the challenges you have been facing and apply His truths to those. Take the time to do some truth journaling, countering little-t truths or outright lies with Big-T truths. Remember to thank God for the hope and encouragement He brings you!

5. **Look Ahead:** What do you have going on the rest of the day? The rest of the week? Think through your hours and upcoming events as best you can. What challenges with food and eating might arise? What difficult, emotional situations might come up? Recount your God-given boundaries and thank God for them. Agree with Him that His boundaries for you truly *have* "fallen for you in pleasant places." Discuss with Him how you might prepare for any

challenging times and be victorious in them. Plan your next appointment with God, whether it be for an hour, half hour, ten minutes, or "on the fly."

6. **Who am I?** End your time reminding yourself of who you are in Christ. For example, "Thank you, Jesus, for choosing me to be Your child. Thank you that I am fearfully and wonderfully made, that I am fully redeemed and forgiven, that I am Your beloved, Your precious one, and that I am always in Your presence and covered by Your grace!"

HALF-HOUR PLAN:

1. **Set the Stage:** Choose a cozy spot in your home, a park bench under a shady tree, a short walk in the park, or it might be a place you know you'll have a half hour or so waiting for someone, like in the car waiting for a child at a music lesson, in a doctor's office waiting room, or at school waiting for a child at a rehearsal. Quiet yourself before the Lord and ask Him to enter into this time with you. Picture Jesus with you right there, wherever you are. (Because He IS!)

2. **Praise and Worship:** Spend a few minutes praising God for who He is. Use your Truth Cards if you have them handy, or a Truth List you keep in your purse or bag. Or, brainstorm aloud the attributes that describe God's character and pray them back to Him. If you have privacy, pray these Big-T truths out loud. If not, pray them quietly in your mind. Another good option is to choose from Sound Cloud files or OriginalThinWithin YouTube videos that might help you renew your mind. (Thin Within sound files are a great resource for your commute to and from work for additional renewing of the mind opportunity!)

3. **Thanksgiving:** Now take a few moments to thank God for the many blessings He has provided you with. Thank Him for the blessings in your current situation. Thank Him for blessings earlier in the day, and those you anticipate later in the day. Be sure to thank Him for your body and the fact that you are fearfully and wonderfully made. Use your Victory List or Gratitude Journal if you have them with you. Otherwise just enjoy giving thanks to your loving King!

4. **Big-T Truth:** If you have your Bible, a devotional, your Truth Cards, or other materials available, use those to fill your mind with God's Big-T Truth. Many participants use praise music in the car, or notes and Scripture on their electronic devices as resources. If no resources are available, say aloud – or think of – memorized Scripture, or recall a few Big-T Truths you learned earlier in your journey. Share with God a specific struggle you have been having and ask Him to help you and provide for you whatever you need from Him in that challenge.

5. **Look Ahead:** Quickly look ahead into your day to spot any challenging situations or emotions that might come up. Ask God to help you come up with a plan for your food and eating so that you will be victorious no matter *what* the circumstances. You might refer to other experiences you have had where you have "observed and corrected" after a misstep.

6. **Who Am I?** End your time with a sentence or two about who you are in Christ. For example, "I am a beloved, valued, and forgiven daughter of God!"

© 2019 Heidi Bylsma, www.renewedlifementoring.com All rights reserved. Printed in the United States of America. No part of this book may be used or reproduced in any matter whatsoever without written permission.

TEN-MINUTE PLAN:

1. **Set the Stage:** Take a deep breath and quiet yourself before the Lord, whether you are at home, on a break at work, in the car, or waiting at a football practice. If you can, close your eyes and just *be* with Him for several seconds. Invite Him into your time together and ask Him to speak His truth and encouragement to your heart.

2. **Praise and Worship:** Lift up your amazing God with one or two sentences about who He is and His glorious character. Do this out loud if you have privacy, or in your mind, if you don't. For example, "Lord, you are mighty to save! You are my refuge and strength. Your power is limitless and nothing is impossible with You! Nothing is too difficult for You! Not even the hardest thing I am dealing with or facing! Your love, mercy, wisdom, and grace are limitless!"

3. **Thanksgiving:** Take a minute to thank God for the blessings that are around you. For example, "Thank You, Jesus, for the gentle snow that is falling outside. … Thank You for these minutes I get to be with You! … Thank you that I am feeling so much better today after struggling with [a sickness]. … Thank You for your provision for my family! … Thank You that your mercies are new every morning, and that it's always morning *somewhere* on Earth!"

4. **Big T Truth:** Bring God's truth into the situation you are in, or one you have been struggling with today. For example: "Lord, I have been waiting in this doctor's office for a long time and my thoughts are full of anxiety. What I know to be true is that You are here with me, You have gone before me, You are protecting me and loving me, and You will provide *whatever* I need!"

5. **Who Am I?** Remind yourself of your rock-solid identity in Christ. For example, "I am a daughter of God and there is nothing that I can't do with His strength within me!" Speak this out loud if you can, or in your mind. One or two sentences will do!

SPONTANEOUS "ON THE FLY!" PLAN:

1. **Setting the stage:** No need! It's already set! *Wherever you are* is the stage, whether you're waiting for a friend to meet you for coffee, doing the dishes, driving to the store, waiting in the car at the school, or taking a shower! *Wherever* you are, He is already there, and is ready and waiting to meet you right where you are at – literally and figuratively! Opportunities to renew your mind "on the fly" come up all day long, *every* day! The key is to *recognize* them and put them to good use. Ask God to help you *redeem* the otherwise-stray and lost moments of your day!

2. **What do you need most right now?** Think this through with the following questions, and connect with God in one of these ways:

    - **Do you need to be reminded of how big and powerful and loving God is?** *Then take a minute to do a quick PraiseFest.*

    - **Do you need to fill your heart with gratitude, to get your mind off of yourself and onto the Lord?** *Spend a minute thanking Him for His blessings.*

© 2019 Heidi Bylsma, www.renewedlifementoring.com. All rights reserved. Printed in the United States of America. No part of this book may be used or reproduced in any matter whatsoever without written permission.

- **Do you need to be reminded of a Big T Truth?** *Choose one and ask God to sink it deeper into your soul, and solidify it in your heart even more.*

- **Do you need to look ahead to ask God to prepare you for what is coming next in your day?** *Ask Him to show you, and then give you, whatever you need to be victorious and peaceful in it.*

- **Do you need to be reminded of who you are in Christ?** *Then tell God who you are. For example, "Lord, I am your girl! You have chosen me and love me more than I can imagine!*

Use these few minutes to renew your mind with *whatever* it is that *you need most* and enjoy the refreshment and peace that God will give you in the midst of your busy day!

APPENDIX B ~ Leader's Guides

This Leader's Guide is intended for a 10-week study of *Thin Within: Fresh Wind Fresh Desire*. The material can be studied in 3 weeks, 6 weeks, 8 weeks, 12 weeks, and 24 weeks. Please modify the study guide to suit your needs for your group.

These notes are only Heidi's rough draft notes—"cheat sheets," really—for leading the online coaching calls each week. You can use her notes to lead an in-person group.

Questions can be posted at a Facebook group set up specifically for this purpose:

https://www.facebook.com/groups/TWFWFDLeaders/

Glossary for this leader guide:

"Meeting" refers to the gathering of people together for the study (either online or in person). It is intended that these meetings be in real time. We recommend establishing a standard that each person will share as you go in order around your "living room" circle. We have done this in live, real-time conference calls with our online meetings. It works well for in-person groups as well.

"Assignment prepared" indicates which lessons the participants have worked through **prior** to the current meeting. It gives a context to the Discussion Questions (see below).

"Discussion Questions participants prepare before coming" ~ These are the questions that will be discussed in the meeting. Please provide these questions to your group members ahead of time so they can prepare. This way, even if they haven't been able to complete the lessons in the assignment, they can nevertheless participate more fully in the group discussion if they prepare their answers to the DQs.

"Notes for meeting" references thoughts or tips, recommendations or considerations you may want to make given the content or structure.

"Assignment for after the meeting" refers to the next assignment that the participants will complete before the NEXT meeting. They begin the work following the meeting and complete it in preparation for the next meeting.

> NOTE: To purchase access to these videos, please contact **support@thinwithinacademy.com**

© 2019 Heidi Bylsma, www.renewedlifementoring.com. All rights reserved. Printed in the United States of America. No part of this book may be used or reproduced in any matter whatsoever without written permission.

Week # ======= Lessons prepared	Discussion Questions participants prepare before coming (and to be asked and discussed in the group meeting).	Notes for meeting	Assignment for after the meeting
01 ===== None (no preparation needed except DQs)	1. What is your name, how long have you been involved with Thin Within, what has your involvement been? How did you hear about Thin Within and what hopes do you have about Fresh Wind, Fresh Desire? 2. What do you hope to experience during the next 10 weeks emotionally, spiritually and physically? 3. As you look at the keys to conscious eating which ones are doable for you? Which ones seem impossible? 4. In the past, when you have committed to releasing weight and keeping it off, what have been your three largest hindrances? What has held you back? 5. Do you have any thoughts as we begin about how you can overcome these hindrances (see #4)? What will it take? Leaders can offer some ideas and brainstorm or ask group members for their input. 6. Please share prayer requests and pray together. 7. Share the assignment for the upcoming week.		**Assignment #1:** 1. Read Intro, Lessons 1, 2, 3 for meeting #02, pages 3 - 18. If you have purchased access to the videos or audios that correspond with this workbook, please view the preview videos that go with the Introduction, and lessons 1, 2 and 3. 2. Please bring your bible and workbook with you to the meetings each week. 3. *God IS doing a new thing… You have NEVER been here before with this group of people doing THIS. This is PROOF that God is doing a new thing. Today, tell yourself this truth again and again… "God is too doing a NEW THING in me!"*

© 2019 Heidi Bylsma, www.renewedlifementoring.com All rights reserved. Printed in the United States of America. No part of this book may be used or reproduced in any matter whatsoever without written permission.

| 02
 =====
 Intro, 1, 2, 3 | 1. What victory have you experienced this week? No victory is too small and insignificant. (Give examples for them to get ideas.)

 2. At the bottom of page 8, we issue a challenge to wait for physical hunger. What is your hunger signal like? Have you noticed anything affecting your recognition of your hunger signal? What are you learning?

 Anyone have a perfect week? Probably not! Our weeks didn't go perfectly and they never will!

 It just isn't going to happen. In Thin Within, we don't let "failure" define us. Instead, we use an observation and correction "tool." Explain 0 and C. We also call it Lessons Learned List.

 Grace abounds….instead of the typical diet….no beating ourselves up. Only learning. God REDEEMS!

 Discuss what the "Lessons Learned List" is (observations lead to corrections. The corrections are the lessons learned.)

 3. What is one observation you have made in the past week about a "mess up" you experienced? What lesson has God been teaching you and what changes are you encouraged you to make? If you aren't sure, we will gladly help out!

 What are your thoughts after you have had a week in our *Thin Within: Fresh Wind Fresh Desire* group, time with the lessons…any questions? Experiences that you want to talk about? Anything meaningful to you? Where did God meet you? Questions?

 4. On page 11 we have you fill in a chart that is the beginning of what we call a God List throughout the FWFD curriculum. Let's go around our circle and share what we gleaned from this activity. | **Assignment #2:**

 1. Complete lessons 4,5, and 6, pages 19-33. If you have purchased access to the videos or audios that correspond with this workbook, please view the preview videos that go with lessons 4, 5, and 6.

 2. Post prayer requests.

 3. Consider blogging your journey complete with "Before, During, and After" Pictures.

 4. This week we will continue to learn about Big T and little t truths and lies. Also, we will look more closely at FAILURE. And BOUNDARIES.

 5. This week, keep a **"Lessons Learned List"** – when you mess up, ask God to show you what you can learn so that you can be equipped for victory. He will redeem the mess up and show you alternative considerations to avoid a mess up and ensure a win! |

| 02
=====
Intro, 1, 2, 3
(Continued) | 5. ACCOUNTABILITY POINTS – Consider emotional, physical, spiritual goals for the next 2 months. An accountability point or a baby step or action step is what we call it when we break down our larger goals into manageable, observable pieces. So, if my goal is to love the Lord more and surrender my eating to him, that is a great goal! But at the end of the day, it is hard for me to know if I have actually done that. So the accountability points that I select should be action items that I know at the end of the day if I have done them or not. (Giving examples of APs for each of my goals is helpful.) Mention that this week is time to consider what APs would be best for you because next week, we will make an assignment of you posting them in Facebook (next week in our call we will ask you to share 2 of them). You will know at the end of the day if you have done it or not. 2, 3, or 4 of them. Preferably only 1 focusing on food and eating. The others on your beliefs. THESE ARE CHANGEABLE…things you wouldn't ordinarily do and need accountability. Checking into the group either daily or 3x each week.

6. PREPARE FOR TRIALS – looking ahead at your week, do you have a potentially challenging situation that you may be facing when your eating boundaries or your commitment to renew your mind is challenged? A house guest? Meeting with difficult people? Spouse out of town? Sick friend or relative? What can you do to prepare yourself so that you can choose victory? Mind renewal? Size of disk? Put fork down? Which person will join you, etc? Truth journal ahead of time? Pull away and renew mind in the bathroom…etc.

7. Please share prayer requests and pray together. | 6. Give some thought and prayer to what Accountability points you can try. Select 2, 3, or 4 specification steps or baby steps, trying to make only one of them focused on food. We have found that people who focus on food and their weight, struggle with experiencing what they hope to during the class. |

03　＝＝＝＝　Lessons 4, 5, 6		**Assignment #3:**

03 — Lessons 4, 5, 6

1. What is one thing that God has encouraged you to do differently this week—a correction or something from your "Lessons Learned List"? Alternatively, share a victory you had this week.

2. What is FAILURE? Discuss failure isn't what we are. It is what we do on occasion. Failure isn't an undertaker, it can be a great teacher. Performance oriented, vs. focusing on Jesus' performance on the cross. Pendulum swing. Get our eyes off of our performance and onto Jesus'.

This is where GOD LIST, Gratitude, Victory List, Praise Fest, lessons learned….all come in. The more we can exalt God and trust him for a work he is doing, the less we will feel like we need to have OUR will, OUR way, OUR eating, OUR food, etc.

3. Do you have any questions about hunger? 0? About satisfaction? 5?

As you continue, you may have begun to notice that you feel emotions more acutely…You get angry more readily. You cry at the drop of a hat. You might even be excessively irritable. If so, CONGRATULATIONS! You are doing it right. No longer numbing with food.

Mind renewal about emotions or about the connection with emotions to food.

Accountability points:

4. What accountability points have you considered incorporating into your journey? How often will you check in? What questions do you have about doing this?

5. In Lesson 4, you wrote down some lies that you have believed. Share One Big T Truth that refutes it (it answers the question "*What does God think about that?*")

6. What is one little t truth you have given too much power? What lie is wrapped up in your previous experience? What Big T Truth refutes this?

7. Please share prayer requests and pray together.

Assignment #3:

1. Please complete Lessons 7, 8, and 9, pages 34-50. If you have purchased access to the videos or audios that correspond with this workbook, please view the preview videos that go with the lessons 7, 8, and 9 as well.

2. Post your APs in our group and check in this week 3x or more.

3. Post a personal prayer request.

04 Lessons 7, 8, 9	1. Share 3 truths from your Truth Cards or Truth Lists	Assignment #4
	Bathroom Scale discussion (Hunger Within pages 85-86) – Options for not being owned by the scale. Friend, starting point, she can tell you up or down and no other weighing, friend keeps your scale, flap over the display, batteries in different place. 2. How do you feel about your relationship with the bathroom scale? (Pages 39 and 40) 3. Upcoming situations, lesson 9 – what situation are you facing? What will you do to live victoriously? 4. Any additional questions about little t truths, lies, and Big T Truths? 5. What are your favorite two God List additions and why? 6. Please share prayer requests and pray together. 7. PRAISE FEST	1. Please complete lessons 10, 11, and 12 on pages 51-64. If you have purchased access to the videos or audios that correspond with this workbook, please view the preview videos that go with the lessons 10, 11, and 12. 2. Please start writing up and adding to your Whole Body Pleasers List and Total Rejects List on pages 56 and 57. 3. Continue to add to your God List. 4. Use Praise Fest during the week to divert your attention away from temptation. Be ready to report to us how it went. 5. Continue to post APs (change them as needed) and check in. Share with us how this is affecting your journey? Can you add anything to your Lessons Learned List?

| 05
===
Lessons 10, 11, 12 | 1. How did it go using a Praise Fest to divert your attention away from a temptation you faced? Did it work?

2. How is it going posting APs and checking in? Are you observing and correcting? Anything you need to ask or suggestions for?

3. How do you feel about eating ANY food? What concerns do you have? What joys?

4. Do you feel like the dieting mentality has a hold on you still? How so? For instance, do you still feel guilty for eating certain foods? Do you still call foods "treats" or "junk?" Are you fearful about gaining weight if you don't exercise? Are you struggling with all or nothing thinking? In what ways are you trying to figure out if the "math" of Thin Within works out compared to counting calories or points? MOST IMPORTANTLY, what BIG T truths does God want you to wall paper your mind with instead of the lies or little t truths that have come from our dieting days?

5. What have you added to your God List from doing page 1 of lesson 12?

6. Share about the Ideal Meal Experience. What plans have you made for your Ideal Meal Experience?

7. Please share prayer requests and pray together. | **Assignment #5:**

1. Complete lessons 15 and 16 on pages 77 - 87. If you have purchased access to the videos or audios that correspond with this workbook, please view the preview videos that go with lessons 10, 11, and 12.

2. Do your "Ideal Meal Experience" if you haven't already. Come ready to tell us about it!

3. Try an old familiar TW tool or a new FWFD tool you haven't tried yet or that you haven't tried in a while. Be ready to share which tool you tried and how it went.

4. Practice the S.T.A.L.L. tool at least 3x this week and share with us how it goes. |

© 2019 Heidi Bylsma, www.renewedlifementoring.com. All rights reserved. Printed in the United States of America. No part of this book may be used or reproduced in any matter whatsoever without written permission.

| 06 **Lessons 13, 14** | 1. Share a victory we can celebrate with you.

2. What was your ideal meal experience like? (page 75) If you told us last week, then share with us what you might try next as an Ideal _____ Experience!

3. Which TW or FWFD tool did you try for the first time or revisit?

4. What did you think about the discussion in lesson 13 about resenting God?

5. How is it going adding to your Whole Body Pleasers, Taste Bud Teasers, and Total Rejects lists?

6. Relative to the discernment phase and exercising more discernment: How do you think being more discerning when eating 0 to 5 will impact you emotionally, spiritually, and physically?

7. Close our time together with a praise fest. Feel free to use what you have added to the charts in the lessons or from your God List. It isn't peeking!

8. Please share prayer requests and pray together. | **Assignment #6:**

1. Complete Lessons 15 and 16 on pages 77-87. If you have purchased access to the videos or audios that correspond with this workbook, please view the preview videos that go with the lessons 15 and 16.

2. If you already tried the Ideal Meal Experience, try the Ideal Ball Game Experience, or the Ideal Movie Experience, or the Ideal Road Trip Experience…or whatever else!

3. Try to pick whole body pleaser foods more frequently. Share with us how that goes. Does it trigger the dieting mentality? Is it freeing? Any challenges? Any blessings? |

| 07 === **Lessons 15, 16** | 1. Please share your victories.

2. In the past 2 weeks, four lessons designed to plunge you in deep to the scriptures to add to your God List. What are your 2 favorite additions to your God List from the material this week? Or…at all. Or…right in this moment what strikes you as being something worth delighting in God's character over.

3. On pages 79 - 80 there is a discussion regarding exercise. Leader or a participant summarizes what TW teaches about exercise.

4. Many of us may need to renew our minds about exercise before we will ever be able to incorporate it into our lives…either because we have previously obsessed or we have always avoided exercise or we think we can't for some reason. What are some lies or little t truths that you struggle with about exercise? What Big T truth can refute these?

5. What activities are you willing to try to incorporate into your life so you can be a bit more active as the Lord directs? (page 81 can give you ideas) (continued below)

6. Have you been successful in using any of the mind renewal tools to change the direction you were headed? Please share it with us. See page 86. | **Assignment #7:**

1. Please complete lessons 17 and 18. If you have purchased access to the videos or audios that correspond with this workbook, please view the preview videos that go with the lessons 17 and 18.

2. Consider creating an "Emergency Kit" or "Survival Kit" – have a basket, box, or spot on your computer or desk for items that you turn to just in those moments when you need an instant bit of help and support. I was given a book of prayers that I have in mine. It is such a great book and so encouraging and I feel God's love in it. I also have "God Speaks to Me" as a devotional and a specific truth list. I also like to include special goodies so that using this Survival Kit is "fun" and encourages me to come to it. Make one and describe it to us. A digital emergency kit… file with links…God List of unique names that minister to you, who I am in Christ list, link to a playlist online or youtube that helps you renew your mind, audio file that you have recorded in your voice memo feature on your phone of your truth cards or something encouraging. |

07 === **Lessons 15, 16 (Continued)**	7. Please share prayer requests and pray together. 8. If time, conclude with a praise fest!	3. Look back over the last 7 weeks. What foods have you had the largest challenge keeping within your 0 to 5 boundaries? Which foods lure you? Be prepared for us to do an exercise together with this. 4. Try a mind renewal tool that you haven't used very often. Evaluate if it is able to help you think God's thoughts after Him. 5. When you are tempted to break your 0 to 5 boundaries or by reaching for a reject or taste bud teaser food, S.T.A.L.L. for a moment (Stop Turn Ask Listen and Love/ Learn) by asking "What need am I trying to meet by eating this/now? Journal about how doing this affects you.

08 === **Lessons 17, 18**	1. Did you create an emergency kit? What have you included? Did you try it? How did it help? What situation were you facing when you tried using it? What WILL you include and when will you make it if you haven't yet. 2. Use the questions and your answers at the bottom of page 89 to respond: "What little t truths, lies, and decision points have you noticed on the way to the point when you break your food and eating boundaries?" James 1 says that when lust conceives it gives birth to sin…there are steps and stages…a progression…to choosing to turn our tails to God and harden our hearts to his guidance in our choice to eat or not eat. 3. What BIG T Truths can refute these…or what corrections can you incorporate so that you can make a different choice at those decision points? 4. What is the difference between shame/guilt and conviction? See page 96. 5. How can you relate to the guilt/shame/overeating cycle? 6. What will you do to break out of this cycle? Mind renewal is the only sure-fire way. Be specific to make a plan to renew your mind about whatever is a source of shame for you. What will you do? When? 7. Use the questions and your answers at the bottom of page 114. to respond: "What little t truths, lies, and decision points have you noticed on the way to the point when you break your food and eating boundaries?" James 1 says that when lust conceives it gives birth to sin…there are steps and stages…a progression…to choosing to turn our tails to God and harden our hearts to his guidance in our choice to eat or not eat. 8. What BIG T Truths can refute these…or what corrections can you incorporate so that you can make a different choice at those decision points? 9. Share prayer requests and pray together.	**Assignment #8:** 1. Please complete lessons 19, 20, 21. If you have purchased access to the videos or audios that correspond with this workbook, please view the preview videos that go with the lessons 19, 20 and 21. 2. Continue to add to your Whole Body Pleasers, Total Rejects, Taste Bud Teasers, and Victory lists! 3. Do the plan asked about in question 6. (Be specific to make a plan to renew your mind about whatever is a source of shame for you. What will you do? When?) 4. In lesson 18 we offer some practical tips. Select one of these and try it out and be ready to tell us about it!

| 09 === **Lessons 19, 20, 21** | 1. Please share your victories.

Perfectionism can undermine the victories God has for us on this journey. It is part of our performance oriented culture and focus on ourselves as the ones who need to "hold it all together."

2. In lesson 19 we asked how perfectionism has been a stumbling block to you in the past and which Big T Truth you can take with you going forward so that it won't dictate victory or defeat?

3. In our last call, we highlighted the shame/guilt cycle. We pointed out that the only way out of this cycle is renewing our minds about what causes us to feel shame. Did you renew your mind about a source of shame that you identified having had in your life? What did you try? Did you notice any difference? Or do you anticipate that, as you continue this process over time, it may have a positive effect on you?

4. Did you Plan to land on "0" at a certain time? How did you do? You might want to observe and correct and do this a couple of times, making improvements each time! Different foods sustain us differently. One of the misunderstandings is that each meal is eaten all the way to a 5. This is not the best approach for most of us as we will eat too much and call it a 5 and also we will not get hungry as often and this can cause us to want to break our boundaries if we want to eat something.

5. Did you try one of the strategies on pages 107 and 108? Which one and how did it go? OR which one will you try this week?

6. See the chart in Lesson 20. The chart is like an "advanced level" observation and correction chart. Share with us about one event, the lies or little t truths you believed, decision points leading up to the event, and the wisdom for next time.

7. Preparation for Trials exercise is on page 116. Share anything that came of this exercise.

8. Gratitudes will be shared around our living room circle. | **Assignment #9:**

1. Please complete lessons 22, 23, and 24. If you have purchased access to the videos or audios that correspond with this workbook, please view the preview videos that go with these lessons.

2. Acquaint yourself with the Appendix in Fresh Wind Fresh Desire. Try one of the Mind Renewal Recipes! Share about it with us. |

10 === **Lessons 22, 23, 24**	1. Lets share victories. But lets do it as a "thank you God for…" a gratitude given to God for being at work in you. 2. Which of the Mind Renewal Recipes did you try? Share with us. 3. What are three lessons learned that God has taught you during this coaching session? These may be corrections you learned as you observed and corrected. 4. In lesson 22, I speak about my story when I was at my worst. Have you ever been in that place? We ask you to share in the What Is Your Story section? What came of this exercise for you? Discuss Modified boundaries…getting rid of one food or another…for how long and "reupping." 5. Refer to Christina's maintenance list in lesson 23. Which of these seems most elusive to you? Which is within your reach? Leader discusses margin of 5. 6. What has God been doing in your life through our study over the past weeks?	

APPENDIX C ~ 8 KEYS TO CONSCIOUS EATING

1. Eat only when my body is hungry.

2. Reduce the number of distractions in order to eat in a calm environment.

3. Eat when sitting down.

4. Eat when my body and mind are relaxed.

5. Eat and drink the food and beverages my body enjoys.

6. Pay attention to my food while eating.

7. Eat slowly and savor each bite.

8. Stop before my body is "full."

© 2019 Heidi Bylsma, www.renewedlifementoring.com All rights reserved. Printed in the United States of America. No part of this book may be used or reproduced in any matter whatsoever without written permission.

APPENDIX D ~ LOOK and LEARN/OBSERVE and CORRECT

As long as we walk this earth, we will be people in process. It is vital to recognize this—especially when we are earnest to learn how to bring our eating under God's leadership. In Thin Within and *Fresh Wind, Fresh Desire*, we encourage you that God can redeem anything! **The only real failure is the failure we fail to learn from.** We won't let failure to define us. Instead, we use the observation and correction tool or what FWFD calls "Look and Learn."

Bathe this entire process in prayer. It can be helpful to journal through it, but it isn't necessary.

FIRST, I will *dispassionately* view what I did that didn't work in accomplishing my godly goals. I want to dismantle the event, *prayerfully* asking God to show me what caused me not to do what I had hoped to do.

Maybe:

- I didn't renew my mind at all today,
    - I didn't wait for hunger.
    - I didn't stop at "just enough"

I go a bit further, by evaluating things like:

- Was I well rested?
- Was I emotional? If so, what was going on?
- Was an "unsafe" person present?
- Had I had too much coffee or tea, causing me to be anxious?
- Had I had a glass of wine, causing me to be less committed to my boundaries?

SECOND, I invite God to show me what lessons I can learn from dismantling this experience or what corrections I can make for the future. As I prayerfully look back with Him, what does He want me to do differently the next time I face a similar situation? Things like:

- Is there a mind renewal tool I can use to be prepared?
- Do I need to go to bed earlier in the evening to be sure I have enough rest?
- Do I need to have boundaries about who I have a meal with?

I do best when I write what the Lord teaches me down in a notebook or journal in a Lessons Learned List.. Then I have a place recording targeted wisdom from Him. A great mind renewal tactic is gratitude and I can thank Him for giving me these Lessons Learned.

Here are some examples from my own Look and Learn list:

© 2019 Heidi Bylsma, www.renewedlifementoring.com. All rights reserved. Printed in the United States of America. No part of this book may be used or reproduced in any matter whatsoever without written permission.

- Keep from having *both* Oreo cookies and vanilla ice cream in the house at the same time until a future date. (This is the lesson I learned when I had an Oreo milkshake for almost every 0 to 5 meal for a couple of days and felt terrible for it.)
- Renew my mind before running errands in town. (This is the lesson learned when I developed a habit of thinking "I deserve to stop at the drive through" because I live in the country far from any fast food!)
- In order to prevent night-time eating, I need to renew my mind about night-time eating between 4pm and 5pm each day and once more for a quick minute immediately following dinner.
- To prevent sinking into emotions of sadness in the evenings, create an "Emergency Kit" filled with resources that I am eager to take time with such as a favorite devotional book, Who I Am in Christ list, Christian Women's Coloring Book, and colored markers.
- Plan activities immediately following dinner that take me out of the house, away from the kitchen. I can take a hot bath (hard to eat in the bathtub), go for a walk, call a friend or relative to encourage her.
- Be cautious about having any alcoholic beverage at all, even with a meal. It is best for me to abstain as it causes me to lose my resolve to keep my eating boundaries.
- I need to renew my mind with one of the mind renewal tools each morning to experience sustained victory on my journey. Take the time, even if it is only 15 minutes.
- Use drive time in the car to renew my mind out loud by speaking a prayer to God of "What is True."

I hope this gives you ideas of how you can actually experience the redemption of your mess-ups, mistakes, and failures. If we learn three things from each mess-up, just think how smart we will be!

Come visit us at **https://www.thinwithin.org/fwfd/** for more resources and information for your journey through *Thin Within: Fresh Wind, Fresh Desire!*

© 2019 Heidi Bylsma, www.renewedlifementoring.com. All rights reserved. Printed in the United States of America. No part of this book may be used or reproduced in any matter whatsoever without written permission.

Made in the USA
San Bernardino, CA
15 July 2019